Health and Healthcare in Complexity

Sandra Jones • Dein Vindigni OAM
Editors

Health and Healthcare in Complexity

3P Ecosystems for Collaborating, Adapting and Leading Change

Springer

Editors
Sandra Jones
College of Business and Law
RMIT University
Melbourne, VIC, Australia

Dein Vindigni OAM
STEM College
RMIT University
Melbourne, VIC, Australia

ISBN 978-981-96-0514-9 ISBN 978-981-96-0515-6 (eBook)
https://doi.org/10.1007/978-981-96-0515-6

This Springer imprint is published by the registered company Springer Nature Singapore Pte Ltd.
The registered company address is: 152 Beach Road, #21-01/04 Gateway East, Singapore 189721, Singapore

I, Sandra, dedicate this book to the many people who have walked beside me as I journey through my life. It begins with my sister Christine, whose untimely death taught me from an early age to look, listen and learn. I trust that her spirit which has accompanied me is content with the pathways we took. Second is my father and mother who taught me it's ok to 'swim against the tide' as long as you have the knowledge to support your views. To my daughters, Aislinn and Kelsey, and husband, Andrew, who each approach the complex world we live in with purpose, passion, integrity, kindness and 'pure guts'. To my colleague, Marina Harvey, who has shared and supported my research journey. To the many students who have walked with me, opening my mind to new knowledge from their experiences, especially Jackie McCann, Ahmed Al Moussa, Jacqueline Pirotta, Cara Kwok and Heather Davis. Finally, to my friend, colleague and co-author, Dein Vindigni, whose dedication and commitment to those living in disadvantage is unwavering. His kindness and perseverance continues to enhance the life of many, including myself.

I, Dein, dedicate this book to the many inspiring companions who have shaped my life's journey to whom I am deeply grateful, including my mother and father who taught me to believe in my dreams and the ability to realise them. To my wife, Catherine, my best friend, greatest supporter and most profound inspiration who has walked every step of life's joys and challenges since we first met. To my children, Daniel and Chiara, who continue to uplift us and bring purpose and joy to our lives. To the beautiful, transformative friendships that bring renewed hope and healing into our lives. To Uncle Paul Gordon, Uncle Paul Callaghan, Aunty April Clarke and all the First Nations friends and mentors who have generously shared their stories enriched by the profound, Ancient Wisdoms of their ancestors. They teach of our connection to all of creation, to love our place and everything in our place and to care for the great gift of Mother Nature for generations to come. These Ancient Wisdoms as passed on by Elders and Ancestors embody the principles of holistic, collaborative partnerships for creating, nurturing and sustaining health and healthcare in a world that so desperately needs to embrace their teachings in order to survive and flourish. To my friend, mentor and distinguished colleague Sandra Jones who has a life-long commitment to challenging linear, hierarchical thinking and promoting justice, equality, holistic health and healthcare. Sandra continues to champion the challenging cause of replacing linear, hierarchical thinking with ecosystem approaches and collaborative partnerships that truly empower individuals and organisations.

Together, we, Dein and Sandra, dedicate this book to our readers, current and future participants in healthcare, who are prepared to accept the challenge of functioning in the ambiguous complex world that is ours. Our hope is that you may draw on the learnings of those who have generously shared their knowledge, insights and practical wisdoms with the courage, passion and purpose to confront the grand challenges of health and healthcare confronting society. To those who dare to care with a vision and commitment to implement a holistic ecosystem to address the complex challenges facing humanity.

Foreword by Anna Ryan

There are countless challenges in the world today, with many of these related to health and healthcare. There are also examples of extraordinary achievements. When reflecting on significant advances, I'm often struck by how many result from a diverse group of people listening to, and learning from, each other with the patient and their needs at the centre. In some instances, this cooperation has emerged through careful planning, but in many instances, it has relied on serendipity.

In contrast, Sandra and Dein's book presents a compelling argument for work to bring about the transformation required in health and health care today. Their premise is that cognitive, operational and relational changes are required to address our contemporary challenges, and they share research findings, practical wisdoms and reflective tools to support this journey.

Skilfully highlighting the inadequacies of Cartesian science, mechanistic thinking and individualist leadership approaches in dealing with today's challenges, Sandra and Dein present a framework merging complexity science and Indigenous wisdoms to embed meaningful collaboration with patients and across professions into our work. Their intentional focus on patient groups most in need of better care, and the collaborative projects used as examples in the later chapters of this book, serves to demonstrate the value of their new paradigm.

This book has been written for those involved in health and health care across all levels and has much to offer practitioners, researchers, educators, health care leaders and policy makers. It will also resonate deeply with patients and with those who care for them. The reflective prompts and the self-reflective templates encourage us to fully engage with the material and to learn from our experiences, to amplify our successes, and to continue to work towards our shared goals of improving health and healthcare for all patients.

Department of Medical Education
Melbourne Medical School
Faculty of Medicine Dentistry & Health Sciences
University of Melbourne
Melbourne, VIC, Australia

Anna Ryan

Foreword by Barry Judd

While disadvantage negatively impacts all aspects of contemporary Indigenous life, it is in the realm of health and healthcare that the persistent suffering of Indigenous people becomes most obvious and the imperative for effective solutions be found the most urgent. Few readers of scholarly works that engage with health and healthcare would have awareness of Indigenous knowledge systems and wisdoms or of their direct applicability to improve the health and well-being of everyone. Medicalised approaches to health and healthcare are rarely questioned due to the improvements in health and healthcare that Western science-based medicine has delivered to billions of people worldwide. Popular understandings that position Western scientific medicine as the only pathway to good health and healthcare have functioned to obfuscate broader understandings of science and medicine as well as definitions of health and healthcare that exist beyond discourses of science and technical medical intervention. In the age of the Anthropocene where global climate change, ecological collapse and diminished social cooperation and cohesion characterise life on earth, the importance of listening to the wisdom of Indigenous peoples' knowledge has never been more urgent.

This book is an important scholarly intervention that helps broaden our understandings of health and well-being and how these might be considered as something that extends far beyond the technical and scientific approach embodied by the Western medical approaches to overcoming poor health and healthcare. It does so through the very deliberate decision to include chapters that focus on understandings of health and healthcare that have emerged from the learnings of Indigenous peoples and their systems of knowledge and wisdom that reach back into antiquity. Authors Uncle Paul Gordon, Uncle Paul Callaghan, Dein Vindigni OAM and Sandra Jones point readers to the possibility of learning from the wisdom of Indigenous Elders and then provide frameworks to cojoin complexity science and ancient wisdom, thereby succeeding in opening new views of health and healthcare that emerge from tried and tested knowledge systems developed and existing beyond the confines of Western science-based medicine. These chapters provide a practical framework for healthcare workers, advocates and decision-makers to consider health and healthcare in a way that is connected to the good health and care of the world. To all who read them I encourage you to listen carefully to the messages about humility, respect and connection; and most of all, I encourage you to reflect on these important learnings and consider how your own approaches and understanding of health and healthcare might be enhanced by referencing the ancient wisdoms to be found in Indigenous knowledge systems.

University of Melbourne
Melbourne, VIC, Australia

Barry Judd

Preface

The aim of this book is to explore the many and various changes required to support health and healthcare[1] to function effectively in a complex world. The underlying premise is that collaboration is fundamental to achieve the extent of cognitive, operational, relational and leadership change required.

Our Journey

This book is the result of a collaborative endeavour between the two authors and the many people who contributed to discussions along the way. Our journey commenced in 2016 when the two authors met at a leadership development training event. At the time, Dr. Dein Vindigni OAM was the Head of the Chiropractic Program in the School of Health and Biomedical Sciences within the College of Science, Technology, Engineering and Mathematics. Professor Sandra Jones was the Director of the Centre for Business Education Research in the College of Business and Law. These form two of the three colleges (the third being the College of Design and Social Practice) of an international university of technology, design and enterprise which is located globally with major sites in Australia, Europe and Asia.

Reflecting on the leadership training, Sandra and Dein shared their concern that it was dominated by a traditional, single leader-centric, hierarchical approach. While there was mention of 'engagement', the focus of the training was on how to become better leaders from positions of power by developing skills and behaviours to lead and manage followers. It presumed a top-down, prescriptive, one-directional flow of communication and information sharing. This was despite considerable research into the contribution of expertise of many that characterises a distributed leadership approach for higher education in which Sandra had been engaged for

[1] We are using the terms health and healthcare as inclusive terminology for a holistic approach.

over 10 years on behalf of the university.[2] Further discussion of their (each) over 35 years experiences led Dein and Sandra to recognise a similar hierarchical approach to leadership in the healthcare sector. This was at odds with their personal common commitment to inclusive leadership for collaboration. Given their eclectic experience (in practice and research), Dein's in clinical healthcare, particularly in Indigenous Health, Aged Care and community-based healthcare and rehabilitation for people experiencing poverty, loneliness and isolation and Sandra's in employment relations, leadership, knowledge management and Complexity science, they decided to engage in a research partnership. The aim was to explore the contribution of collaboration (and leadership for collaboration) that would assist health and healthcare to become a complex adaptive system capable of operating in the complex world. In turn, this led to their decision to author a book designed to demonstrate a holistic ecosystem of health and healthcare in which the importance of collaboration is highlighted.

This book is designed to present the breadth of issues to be considered, rather than an in-depth discussion of each issue. References are provided at the end of each chapter for readers wishing to engage at greater depth. The chapters explore a conjoining of philosophies, fields of research and Ancient Indigenous Wisdoms to enable adaptation that includes the most relevant aspects of each. Most importantly, this book is designed to assist self-identification, by individuals and groups, of actions for change that are suited to their context and culture. To this end, this book provides a suite of four resources, as self-enabling reflective templates, each with a series of reflective prompts.

Collaborating Along the Journey

In journeying along our collaboration path, and in order to 'practice what we preach', we adopted the 6 tenets of a distributed leadership approach[3] to underpin our co-design, co-creation and co-writing of this book as follows:

1. We *enabled* a context and culture of trust and respect by circulating an overview of the aim of this book to people who expressed a similar commitment.
2. We *engaged* a diverse range of experts from a cross section of health and healthcare disciplines with experience in collaborative partnerships for healthcare.
3. We *enacted* processes and support to encourage ongoing participation using face-to-face and digital mediums.
4. We *encouraged* participation and collaboration through ongoing communication of ideas as they emerged and organised a webinar to share ideas.
5. We *evaluated* the effectiveness of our collaboration through ongoing opportunities for feedback and peer review.

---

[2] Jones 2017, 2020; Jones and Harvey 2017; Jones et al. 2012, 2014

[3] See Chap. 10 for further explanation.

6. We encouraged *emergence* of ideas, understandings and new knowledge through an iterative process.

Methodology

In seeking to choose a methodology appropriate for the argument presented in this book, and at the same time ensure we adopted a research approach that is inclusive of disciplinary approaches and of Western and Indigenous cultures, we chose a reflective practice methodology. This is explained more clearly in Part III that also includes a detailed literature review and analysis.

Melbourne, VIC, Australia Sandra Jones
Melbourne, VIC, Australia Dein Vindigni OAM

References

Jones S (2017) Leading the Academy: Distributed leadership in higher education. HERDSA Guide. HERDSA Sydney. ISBN 9780994554642.

Jones, S (2020) Distributed leadership. In David M.E, Amey M.J (eds) SAGE encyclopedia of higher education: 378–381, Thousand Oaks: SAGE Publications.

Jones S, Harvey M (2017) A distributed leadership change process model for higher education, Journal of Higher Education Policy and Management, Special Edition: Leading the Academy, Building Capacity for Distributed Leadership: 26–139 https://doi.org/10.1080/1360080X.2017.1276661

Jones S, Harvey M, Lefoe G, Ryland K (2012). Lessons learnt: identifying synergies in distributed leadership projects: Final report. Office for Learning and Teaching. Retrieved from https://ltr.edu.au/resources/LE9_1222_Jones_Report_2012_0.pdf. Accessed 16 Mar 2024.

Jones S, Hadgraft R, Harvey M, Lefoe G, Ryland K (2014) Evidence-based benchmarking framework for a distributed leadership approach to capacity building in learning and teaching. https://ltr.edu.au/resources/LE11_2000_Jones_Report_2014_0.pdf. Accessed 16 Mar 2024.

Acknowledgements

The authors acknowledge the challenges, for all participants, inherent in adopting a collaborative approach. These challenges, particularly from competing work and time demands, were experienced in the preparation of this book. This led to continual experimentation with approaches to engaging experts in discussions. It did result in the final chapters' preparation being undertaken by fewer authors than we had initially supposed, however, we acknowledge the input of ideas, knowledge and experience from a wide range of people. We would like to express our heartfelt thanks to all those who provided ideas, knowledge and experience and who contributed to the iterative review process. While the authors of the chapters take full responsibility for the final written outcome, we would like to express our gratitude to the many individuals who provided their thoughts, ideas, reflections and proposals for change, including Kerryn Butler-Henderson; Regina Crameri; Aunty Kerrie Doyle; Marina Harvey; Peter Hayes; Andries Kleynhans OAM; Noel Lythgo; (the late) Peter McLean; Kirsty Marles; Peta Phelan; Prasad Podugu; Jenny Robinson; Jacinta Ryan; and David Spillman.

The authors would like to extend their gratitude to the two proof editors, Laura E Goodin and Ann Raybould, for their untiring attention to detail that resulted in immeasurable improvement to the prose and flow of the chapters.

Reviews

A collaborative review process was employed, combining iterative feedback from many people, including those identified above, with editorial feedback and an academic blind review process. Special thanks go to the authors who reviewed chapters and to Heather Davis, Bernardo Figueiredo and David Spillman.

Contents

Notes on Contributors

Salma Arabi, an emerging academic in digital health, is dedicated to unravelling the complexities of healthcare access and equity. As a lead researcher at RMIT University and Head of Discipline, Digital Health at Charles Sturt University, she actively contributes to digital health partnerships. Her commitment extends to exploring the intricate challenges of healthcare accessibility. As a translational scientist, Salma uniquely bridges the gap between theory and practice. Her expertise signifies a profound understanding of disparities within healthcare, emphasising a commitment to substantive contributions that advance both academic discourse and practical applications in the evolving field of digital health.

Brian Budgell is a Canadian biomedical researcher with a special interest in the languages of biomedicine and health. During his 14 years as a resident researcher in Japan, he travelled extensively throughout East Asia and Australia, facilitating inter-institutional collaborations and conducting studies on intra- and interprofessional communications. Since 2009, he has been a director of Global Peace Network, a Canadian-registered charity that focuses on improving physical rehabilitation in East Africa through direct patient care and continuing professional education.

Uncle Paul Callaghan is an Aboriginal man from the land of the Worimi, coastal New South Wales, Australia. He uses his lived experience, cultural and community knowledge, experience as a CEO of a training organisation with an annual budget of $60 million, studies in commerce and PhD in Creative Practice to advise organisations on how to implement strategic transformation initiatives that will increase the effectiveness of services targeting Aboriginal peoples. He is also a best-selling and award-winning author, along with Uncle Paul Gordon, of a book titled *The Dreaming Path* that provides insights into traditional Aboriginal ways of knowing, being and doing and how they can be used by all people to achieve improved well-being individually and globally.

Uncle Paul Gordon is a Ngemba man, born in Brewarrina, a small town located on the Barwon River, northwestern New South Wales. Since 1983, he has spent a lot of his time with Old Men, performing cultural activities and learning Aboriginal Lore. His passion is to keep traditional Aboriginal ceremony alive as he sees it as an important part of the well-being of Aboriginal people today. Uncle Paul has been a CEO of an Aboriginal training organisation where his leadership model included the incorporation of cultural values into mainstream business practices. He recently completed a Master of Philosophy degree. Today, he is recognised as a senior Elder and is one of the highest initiated Aboriginal men in New South Wales.

Sandra Jones is a Professor Emerita in the School of Management at RMIT University in Australia. Sandra has spent over 35 years researching and teaching across an eclectic field of studies, including leadership, employment relations, Complexity sciences and knowledge management. Sandra has been professionally engaged across a broad range of industries and organisations, including education and health, in both the private and public sectors, nationally and internationally. Sandra is deeply committed to the value of collaboration in order to respond to, adapt and lead change in the complex world. She is an acknowledged international expert in Distributed Leadership and educational design for professional practice.

Ashleigh Moreland is a dynamic and accomplished neuroscientist, author, speaker, therapist, consultant and supervisor of research students. She has a PhD in neuroplasticity, a passion for bridging the gap between scientific inquiry and real-world application and a vision for leveraging emerging technologies and innovative clinical modalities to improve access and outcomes for complex issues globally. Ashleigh founded the Re-MIND Institute, through which she delivers programmes worldwide to improve emotional, mental, physical, relational and spiritual well-being.

Barbara Polus is a Principal Research Fellow, School of Engineering, RMIT University. She works as a team member on projects that develop affordable diagnostic tools for people with neurodegenerative diseases living in rural and remote communities. She served as the CEO of the not-for-profit organisation 'Hands-on-Health Australia' from 2012 to 2017. Prior to that she was a director and volunteer of the organisation, where she initiated the first RMIT University chiropractic student clinic at the Sacred Heart Mission, Hands on Health Clinic. She has worked collaboratively to develop and implement train-the-trainer programmes for managing musculoskeletal conditions in developing countries, including Timor-Leste, Indonesia and the Philippines.

Dein Vindigni OAM is a chiropractic practitioner with over 30 years of private practice experience. Since 2015, Dein has converted his practice-based experience into academic research and teaching in the School of Health and Biomedical Sciences at RMIT University. Throughout his career, Dein has been actively involved in providing voluntary health care, and in 1987, he founded the organisation Hands-On-Health Australia (HOHA). Dein continues to volunteer his expertise in the provision of Allied and Complementary Healthcare and clinical training programmes for underserved communities. Dein's primary research contributions focus on Indigenous Health, Aged Care and community-based healthcare and rehabilitation for people experiencing poverty, loneliness and isolation.

Abbreviations

ABS	Australian Bureau of Statistics
ACHS	Aboriginal Community Health Service
AHAH	Aboriginal Health in Aboriginal Hands
AHP	Adaptive Health Practice
AHS	Aboriginal Health Service
AMS	Aboriginal Medical Service
ANT	Actor Network Theory
AHW	Aboriginal Health Workers
AR	Action Research
AIATSIS	Australian Institute of Aboriginal and Torres Strait Islander Studies
CAS	Complex Adaptive Systems
CARE	Collaborative Adaptive Resilient Ecosystem
CAG	Community Advisory Group
CD	Capacity Development
CEO	Chief Executive Officer
CRA	Collaborative Research Agreements
CoI	Community of Interest
CORE	Cognition, Organisation, Relationships, Engagement
DARE	Distributive Action Relational Ecosystem
EBD	Evidence-Based Practice
ECHO	Extension for Community Healthcare Outcomes
DHHRP	Digital Health Hub Rehabilitation Project
FWA	Family Wellbeing Empowerment
HAF	Health Access Framework
HBM	Health Belief Model
HEARS	The Health Ecosystem Action Relationship for Sustainability
HESJF	Health Equity and Social Justice Framework
HoH	Hands on Health
IHCP	Informal Healthcare Providers
IHC	Integrative Healthcare
IPE	Interprofessional Education

LEADS	Lead Self; Engage Others; Achieve Results; Develop Coalitions; Transform Systems
LEAP	Lead(er)ship Ecology of Adaptive Practice
LGBTQ+	Lesbian, Gay, Bisexual, Transgender, Queer, Intersex, Agender and Asexual
LLL	Living Learning Lab Pty Ltd.
LMIC	Low-Middle Income Countries
MoU	Memorandum of Understanding
NFP	Not-For-Profit
NHS	National Health Service (UK)
OECD	Organisation for Economic Co-operation and Development
PAR	Participatory Action Research
PCC	Patient-Centred Care
PP	Patients as Partners
PHA	Pathways to Healthy Ageing
PHC	Primary Health Care
PREM	Patient-Reported Experience Measures
PROM	Patient-Reported Outcomes Measures
RACF	Residential Aged Care Facility
RCC	Relationship-Centred Care
THTDP	Transnational Health Training Digital Partnership
SDHF	Social Determinants of Health Framework
SEER	Self-Enabling Ecosystem for Reflection
SNA	Social Network Analysis
STTEP	Sustainable Training, Treatment, Employment Program
UN	United Nations
WHO	World Health Organization
3Ps	Principles and Purposes; People in Place; Practices and Processes
6Es	Engage, Enable, Enact, Encourage, Evaluate, Emergent
6Ls	Lore, Love, Look, Listen, Learn, Lead (or Leave alone)

List of Figures

List of Tables

List of Templates

Part I
Change in Health and Healthcare: Why a Paradigm Shift?

Part I of this book seeks to establish the reasons for advocating a paradigm change for health and healthcare as a holistic ecosystem. The first two chapters (Chaps. 1 and 2) summarise the impact of Cartesian science on health and healthcare that has led to a separation of professions, of professionals and patients and the institutionalization of hierarchies of decision making. Chapter 3 adds the challenge of the lack of a spiritual understanding of the biophilia connection of Indigenous peoples, while Chap. 6 adds the lack of cultural understanding on access and equity to health and healthcare. This Cartesian science influence is contrasted with the needs of health and healthcare based in an understanding of Complexity science. Attempts to change the negative impacts of Cartesian science are discussed in Chaps. 4 and 5 however it is concluded that these attempts at change have had limited success or impact. In response the authors propose a (re-imagined) paradigm of health and healthcare as a holistic ecosystem that acknowledges the importance of collaboration in cognition, action to build relationships and leadership. To explore this, first, the many influences on health and healthcare are classified as three agencies of health and healthcare: Principles and Purpose (P1), People in Place (P2) and Practices and Processes (P3). Second, a potential conjoining of Cartesian and Complexity science is proposed with the aim of easing the transition from one paradigm to another. A second potential conjoining of Complexity science and Ancient Indigenous Wisdoms is discussed in (Chap. 13) in Part II.

Chapter 1
Introduction

Sandra Jones and Dein Vindigni OAM

Abstract The focus of this chapter is to establish the purpose of the book. It presents the challenges for health and healthcare arising from the increasingly complex context in which health and healthcare operate. It highlights the difference between cognition, action and leadership based in the principles of Complexity and Cartesian science. It promotes the re-imagining of health and healthcare as a holistic ecosystem that acknowledges three agencies of health and healthcare: Principles and Purposes (P1); People in Place (P2); and Practices and Processes (P3), and the importance of interconnections between these agencies. Each of the issues identified are discussed in more detail in the chapters in Part I.

1.1 What Is This Book About and Why Is It Important? Complexity Facing Health and Healthcare

Studies of Complexity science have highlighted that to accept that the world is complex, rather than predictable and controllable, is to "change our approach to everything: our approach to change, to management, to policy development, to evaluation, to leadership and to living" (Boulton et al. 2015, p. 123). Complexity consists of many interacting elements (agencies) that coevolve with the environment and display features of both self-organization and emergence. This requires the replacement of the linear thinking that has accompanied the mechanistic age of Cartesian science, with open systems thinking that accompanies Complexity science. It also

S. Jones (✉)
Business and Law College, RMIT University, Melbourne, VIC, Australia

D. Vindigni OAM
STEM College, RMIT University, Melbourne, VIC, Australia
e-mail: dein.vindigni@rmit.edu.au

S. Jones, D. Vindigni OAM (eds.), *Health and Healthcare in Complexity*,
https://doi.org/10.1007/978-981-96-0515-6_1

requires the need to understand the different ways of thinking between diverse groups. Speaking of Indigenous peoples, Professor Barry Judd[1] states:

> The recent emergence of Complexity science creates the possibility for Ancient Indigenous Wisdoms to inform better understandings of health and better practices of healthcare. This comes at a time when all life on earth is at risk due to unconstrained human activity. In the age of the Anthropocene where global climate change, ecological collapse and diminished social cooperation and cohesion characterise life on earth, the importance of listening to the wisdom of Indigenous peoples' knowledges has never been more urgent. What these knowledges can teach everyone are the fundamental truths that govern sky and earth. This means we humans need to be humble and respectful and caring of all other things we encounter in the world. It also means that a healthy earth requires balance to be maintained in order for our health to be safeguarded, protected and cared for. On the other hand, are the shortcomings of western systems to 'fix' the Indigenous health and healthcare that often escape valid critique and necessary debate about their efficacy to improve outcomes for the better. Medicalised approaches to health and healthcare are rarely questioned due to the improvements in health and healthcare western science-based medicine has delivered to billions of people world-wide. Popular understandings that situated western scientific medicine as the only pathway to good health and healthcare have functioned to obfuscate broader understandings of science and medicine as well as definitions of health and healthcare that exist beyond discourses of science and technical medical intervention. (Personal communication to author 2024)

This book explores the many changes required to adopt a new paradigm of health and healthcare as a holistic ecosystem. The nomenclature heath and healthcare is used throughout this book as an inclusive concept that recognizes that a holistic approach requires change by both individuals living a healthy lifestyle and by healthcare service and support providers. This has become increasingly apparent since the COVID-19 pandemic demonstrated our increasingly complex world. We highlight the need for a holistic ecosystem to identify and promote networks and flows between individuals and processes to increase social learning that helps to shape norms, productivity, and creativity. Pentland (2014, Chap. 3) used the term social physics to explain how the ubiquitous digital data of social learning can be utilised to understand how the flow of ideas turns behaviours into action:

> most of our public beliefs and habits are learned by observing the attitudes, actions and outcomes of our peers, rather than by logic or argument. Learning and reinforcing this social contract is what enables a group of people to coordinate their actions effectively.

The authors are committed to the belief that to treat health and healthcare as if it is predictable and controllable is to contribute to a system that is unable to address current, let along future, needs. We acknowledge that, while there has been discussion of the need for integration and collaboration in health and healthcare between the professions, and between professionals and patients, there are few examples of success. In response, we propose the re-imagining of health and healthcare as a holistic ecosystem that acknowledges three agencies: Principles and Purpose (P1), or the philosophy and reasoning (cognition) that underpins health and healthcare;

[1] Professor of Indigenous Studies and Deputy Vice Chancellor, Indigenous at The University of Melbourne.

People in Place (P2), or the relationships between people and the context and culture in which they are engaged and Practices and Processes (P3), or the actions, systems and support through which health and healthcare is operationalized. Emphasis is placed on the interconnections between the 3Ps, which are characterized as nodes on a tripod in Fig. 1.1.

In proposing a holistic ecosystem of health and healthcare we acknowledge the claim that Cartesian science has maintained its attraction as it appears to provide order, purpose and control, and thus, as Boulton et al. (2015, p. 3), maintained the mechanistic view "seduces us with certainty and a belief in the existence of identifiable causes to identifiable effects when in reality such predictions and certainty rarely exist." In contrast, accepting Complexity science, they claimed, requires us to:

> counter certainty and fixedness in assuming any approach. We are advocating more tentativeness and less hubris. We think that a complexity perspective sits in the middle ground. It suggests 'try and see' or 'try several things and see' rather than 'the analysis of the situation shows this is the right way to tackle it… We need to be wary of assuming everything can be tested and evidenced, and imagining that we can always know what caused what or what might happen next. We need to be more willing to experiment, to fail, and to learn from these failures—without giving up on clarity, and without abandoning the use of concrete data to plan and measure within limits' (Boulton et al. 2015, p. 6)

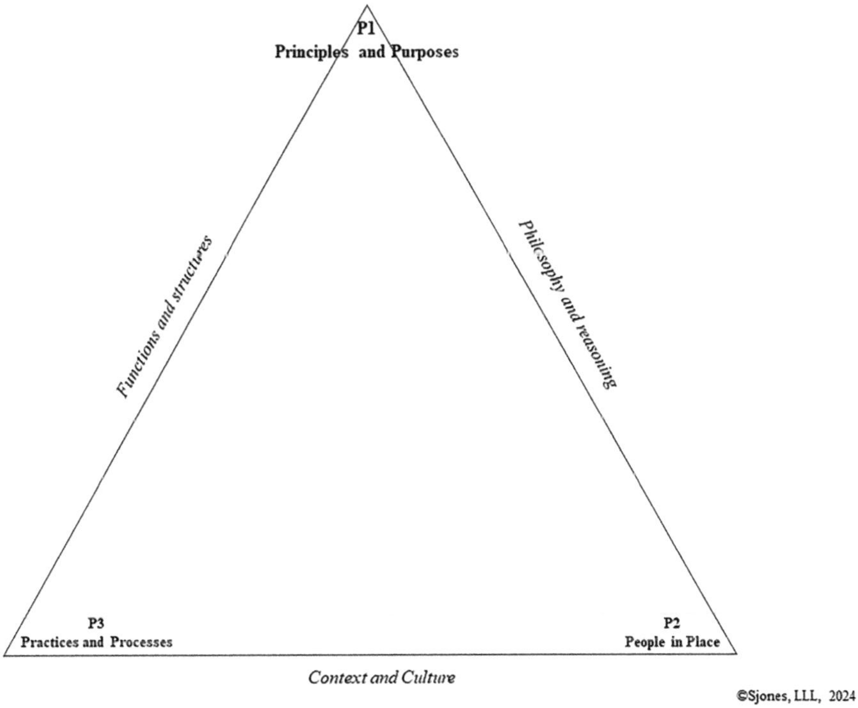

Fig. 1.1 The 3P Agencies of Health and Healthcare

1.2 So, What Should We Do? The Contribution of Collaboration

In exploring the paradigm shift of health and healthcare as a holistic ecosystem, we are committed to challenging many current assumptions. We acknowledge the importance of garnering the knowledge of all experts involved in healthcare: professionals, patients, family, and community. In our case we bring to the discussion expertise in health, organizational theory, leadership and Ancient Indigenous Wisdoms. To ensure a shared understanding we recognise that this requires collaboration to build relationships and commitment to the emergence of new ideas. To this end, the book presents more than simply a discussion of change, or a presentation of models, or a list of 'how to', to do so would have us fall back into the mechanistic trap of assuming singe linear cause and effect. In contrast, our approach echoes the thoughts of an Indigenous Aboriginal Elder[a] that:

> It is not my job to *give* you answers. Aboriginal peoples (the world over) know all too well the pains of being told *your truth is wrong- here take ours*. (Kakkib Li'Dthia Warrawee'a 2002, p. 114)

Through this approach we aim to present a series of signposts designed for those engaged in health and healthcare to navigate along a pathway that suits their context and culture. We adopt what can be described as *wayfaring* that consists of *wayfinding* (navigating, observing and identifying likeness and systems), *wayshowing* (trailblazing, leaving clues, planning and creating new directions), and *waysharing* for greater understanding (storytelling, transferring information, sensemaking and consciously evolving). A wayfaring approach is illustrated by Spiller, Barclay-Kerr, and Panoho (2015, p. 36) in their description of the New Zealand Māori:

> After diligently reading the signs and adjusting yourself as the waka- needle, conceiving yourself as still and becoming calibrated to a moving world, an island appears on the horizon ahead. You keep the island in your mind's eye, but do not try to aim for it in a straight line; rather you continue to adjust to signs, with the world moving past you……Eventually the island comes closer and closer to you and the wake, and then it arrives.

In our case, we, first, observed to identify likenesses through exploring, analyzing and reflecting upon what is currently known and discussed in the literature. Based on our findings, we created new directions for changes in cognition, actions to build relationships and leadership to engage more experts in decision making. This analysis and reflection drew from a range of fields of thought including physics, philosophy, engineering, economics, management, and science, with the aim of identifying interconnections between the knowledge and understanding from these different fields. This resulted in our assemblage of several ecologies to demonstrate the interlinks between the 3P agencies of health and healthcare. These (provided in Part II) are termed as follows:

(i) A Collaborative Adaptive Resilient Ecology (CARE of cognition) (Chap. 8).
(ii) A Distributive Action Relational Ecology (DARE) (Chap. 9).
(iii) A Lead(er)ship Ecology of Adaptive Partnerships (LEAP) (Chap. 10).
(iv) An Action Cognition Ecology of Lead(er)ship (ACEL) for Collaboration (Chap. 10).

Third, we assembled four Self Enabling Ecologies of Reflection (SEER) related to each of the aspects of change considered: Cognition (SEER C); Action to build relationships (SEER A); Lead(er)ship (SEER L); acknowledgement of the Spiritual (through the Ancient Indigenous Wisdoms), (SEER S). The SEERs are designed to assist readers to reflection upon, and analyze change needed to achieve a holistic, ecosystem of health and healthcare.

Fourth, in PIII, we present the findings of reflection-on-practice of the experience of five projects designed as collaborative partnerships to provide integrated health and healthcare. The reflections were assisted by the co-editors, Dein who was directly involved in each project and Sandra with her expertise in reflective practice. By serendipity, the initial focus of each of these projects was in the provision of allied and complementary health that extended overtime to include clinical, general practice, nursing, and physiotherapy. Collaborations were between not-for-profit organizations, professional associations, universities (including students), and individual health professionals and employees of not-for-profit organization. The importance of such collaborations was explained by a palliative care physician and clinical educator, Dr. Terry Hannan (2018, p. viii):

> In my role as a clinical educator I have regularly reminded those I am attempting to educate that anyone caring for an unwell (dis-eased) person, that is clinicians (nurses, doctors, pharmacists etc), are authorised or legally permitted to push, probe, poke, cut, strip naked and poison (medications) other persons while recognising or not recognising the harm we may do. For all of us in these positions we need to recognise and reaffirm that these are indeed profound responsibilities and privileges.

1.3 Why Read This Book?

This book is addressed to all who are seeking ways to address the complexity of current and future health and healthcare. This includes healthcare providers, patients and their families, managers, leaders, policymakers, peak bodies researchers, educators, and student practitioners who acknowledge the need for profound change in response to the complexity facing health and healthcare. It will have immediate resonance for students and new recruits to health and healthcare who recognize the complexity, and ambiguity they face. It presents ideas for how to design innovative futures for practitioners and policy advisors who see the advantage of a forward-looking strength-based approach based in collaboration.

In recognizing the challenge of adopting a new holistic ecosystem of health and healthcare, we have structured the book as follows. First, (Pt I), an overview of the challenges of health and healthcare working in a complex world are discussed. These challenges include the need for change in cognition, action to build relationships, and leadership to engage experts. Issues of access and equity are also explored, with a particular focus on the issues facing Indigenous peoples and people living in lower-income countries. Second, (Pt II), discusses a strength-based approach is adopted to explore the potential for change. This results in the assemblage of several ecologies design to assist changes in modes of cognition, methods of actions to build relationship, and approach to lead(er)ship. Based on these ecologies, four resources are created designed to support changes to build and maintain health and healthcare as a holistic ecosystem appropriate to different contexts and cultures. Part III reflects upon the experience of five projects that aimed to use a collaborative partnership approach to provide integrated health and healthcare to people living in disadvantage. Finally, Part IV presents a proposal for actioning change from 'the edge' through projects.

1.4 Conceptual Considerations

In proposing fundamental change to re-imagine a holistic ecosystem of health and healthcare, we have sought to ensure that, while each chapter can stand alone, we encourage reading the entire book rather than confine reading to individual chapters. This will help develop knowledge and understanding of the proposal from all three agencies of Principles and Purposes; People in Place and Practices and Processes.

The book requires the adoption of a reflexive approach to first consider, and then operationalize, change rather than to rely imposed on regulation. It promotes the value of collaboration, and advocates change that originates with practitioners and students in practice. While this is more demanding than the usual prescribed map of actions imposed from above, the self-reflective approach encourages change that can become embedded and sustained.

1.5 Our Stance

This book is written to encourage a holistic, collaborative approach. It is recognized that this may need to come from 'the edge' rather than from those entrenched in the current paradigm (see Pt. III). This has several aspects:

1. It advocates the adoption of a paradigm shift based in a holistic ecosystem of health and healthcare.
2. It incorporates consideration of the spiritual underpinning of the Ancient Indigenous Wisdoms.
3. It gives voice to the patient and professionals committed to a holistic approach to health and healthcare.
4. It advocates for interprofessional collaboration and education that goes beyond integration to co-development and co-design by professions and patients.
5. It proposes the addition of reflexive practice to add 'learning through doing' to evidence-based-practice.

6. It encourages the development of a self-determining approach rather than a ‘how to’ map with a list of actions.

This combination, while more demanding than simply mapping lists of things ‘to do,’ has the advantage providing opportunities to self-design action in which consideration is given to potential issues before action is taken, thus removing the need for ‘fighting fires’ that could have been avoided.

References

Boulton JG, Allen PM, Bowman C (2015) Embracing complexity: strategic perspectives for an Age of Turbulence, Oxford University Press
Hannan TJ (2018) Bedside stories: a journey built by patients, learning to listen. Manufactured by Amazon.com.au, Sydney
Kakkib li’Dthia Warrawee’a (2002) There once was a tree called Deru / Kakkib li’Dthia Warrawee’a. Thorsons, Pymble
Pentland A (2014) Social physics. Scribe Publications, Brunswick Victoria and Sans Way London
Spiller C, Barclay-Kerr H, Panoho J (2015) Wayfinding Leadership. Huia Publishers, Wellington NZ

Chapter 2
Health and Healthcare in a Complex World: A Paradigm Shift

Sandra Jones and Dein Vindigni OAM

Abstract The focus of this chapter is on providing a detailed explanation of the changes required in health and healthcare to present to the complex world. The aims of this chapter are twofold. First, to present a summary of negative impact of the design of health and healthcare arising from exclusive focus on the principles of Cartesian science. Second, to propose a new (re-imagined) paradigm for health and healthcare as a holistic ecosystem. To explain this holistic ecosystem, the influences on health and healthcare are classified under three agencies of health and healthcare (identified in Chap. 1): Principles and Purposes (P1), People in Place (P2), and Practices and Processes (P3).

2.1 Cartesian-based (Traditional) Paradigm of Health and Healthcare

2.1.1 Principles and Purposes (P1)

The literature suggests that Cartesian science has dominated thinking upon, and actions designed for, health and healthcare in much of the, so-called, developed world (Gislason and Bendelow 2013).[1] Gold (1985, p. 664) described this as assuming an ontology of mankind as "a composite dualism: the separation of mind and body … [with]…. the human body conceived as a purely passive machine driven by

[1] This book includes a series of chapters that discuss what adoption of Ancient Indigenous wisdoms might contribute to a paradigm change.

S. Jones (✉)
Business and Law College, RMIT University, Melbourne, VIC, Australia

D. Vindigni OAM
STEM College, RMIT University, Melbourne, VIC, Australia
e-mail: dein.vindigni@rmit.edu.au

S. Jones, D. Vindigni OAM (eds.), *Health and Healthcare in Complexity*,
https://doi.org/10.1007/978-981-96-0515-6_2

mechanical causality." This mechanistic thinking focuses on analyzing facts, predicting the future, deciding how to intervene, making and executing plans, as well as controlling and measuring outcomes. McDaniel et al. (2013, p. 6) stated that mechanistic thinking applied to mankind is most forcefully represented by Newton's three laws of nature, particularly the second law which explains and allows for "prediction of behaviour of mechanical phenomena on both terrestrial and celestial levels." In health and healthcare, this has led to the body being viewed as a "mechanism with a separation between mind and body…[*with*]….human beings seen as biological organisms (materialism), to be understood by their constituent parts (reductionism), using the principles of anatomy, physiology, biochemistry and physics" (Mehta 2011, p. 204).

Based in this philosophy, the purpose of healthcare has been seen as the removal of disease through the application of medicine (World Health Organization 1946; Hart 1985). In this scenario, healthcare providers are regarded as needing "to be in control" (McDaniel et al. 2013, p. 22).

2.1.2 People in Place (P2)

It is argued that the traditional mechanistic philosophical framework fails to focus on the importance of people in their particular context and culture. Boulton, Allen, and Bowman (2015, p. 3) stated:

> it does not easily lend itself to exploring interrelationships, co-evolution, dynamic flows, values, unintended consequences, multiple perspectives, learning, the emergence of the totally unexpected, collapse, the way differing factors interact – or give sufficient consideration to the distant future or the role of the past.

Mechanistic thinking has resulted in a separation between medical professions and subprofessions, each of which has been bounded by different specialized knowledge, skills, beliefs, values, norms of behavior, routines, traditions, and sensemaking. This has resulted in often skeptical responses by patients to non-biological explanations for their illnesses as unreal, illegitimate, and unscientific (Mehta 2011).[2] It has created a culture in which communication and negotiation is tied to professional identity that has impacted attitudes, beliefs, and perceptions through "memory traces that group members carry with them" (Noyes 2021, p. 68). Given that culture is "one of the most powerful and stable forces operating in organizations" (Schein 1996, p. 231), patterns of care have become similarly separated (Mannion and Davies 2018). The visible manifestation of culture, the physical artifacts, arrangements, and behaviors associated with getting things done, has been described as being "given precedence over developing shared beliefs, values, norms of behavior, routines, traditions, and sensemaking" (Parmelli et al. 2011, p. 2).[3]

[2] Discussed further in Chap. 5.

[3] Discussed further in Chap. 7.

It has presaged technical (surgical) solutions, rather than therapeutic procedures and medications, and has in turn fostered patients' belief that they are simply recipients of technical solutions rather than being participants in their own health as part of adaptive change (Pomey et al. 2015; Thygeson 2013).[4] It has also resulted in separation between Western (mechanistic) and Indigenous (spiritual) approaches to health and healthcare[5] and in lack of understanding of the importance of culture and context contributing to unequal access to healthcare[6].

2.1.3 *Practices and Processes (P3)*

Mechanistic thinking has impacted on the practices and processes implemented in health and healthcare through design based on the assumption of linear, one-directional cause and effect associations, in which events occur sequentially. The biomedical model that accords with a reductionist medicine paradigm has been described as based on action "where a problem is broken down into its smallest components, examined, and then the information gleaned used to draw conclusions about the nature of the larger reality" (Tuffin 2016, p. 349). Each variable within the linear system is assumed to act independently, with output regarded as proportional to input and linkages between cause and effect reproducible over time for any given input (Tuffin 2016). This has enabled clinicians to feel confident in their ability to treat disease "through the examination of physiological principles" (Kurdack 2016, p. 1015).

The biomedical model has also resulted in a hierarchy being established in which physicians "typically remain at the top of the interdisciplinary hierarchies" (Noyes 2021, p. 63). Physicians have been afforded legal and ethical responsibility for patient care, with nonphysicians often excluded from aspects of the patient care process. Ancillary staff whose disciplines are grounded in biopsychosocial or relationship-centered models (such as occupational therapy or spiritual therapy), have not been afforded the same attention (Noyes 2021). Open disagreement of physicians by nonphysicians has been discouraged through the "unspoken rule … that doctors make decisions" (Noyes 2021, p. 67). The result is that healthcare services are "notoriously varied, fractured by speciality, occupational groupings, professional hierarchies, and service lines" (Mannion and Davies 2018). Over time, methods of inquiry based on abstraction that can be measured have become preferred over ethnographic or clinical observation of organizational phenomena (Schein 1996). Evidence-based research (EBR), with its emphasis on 'robust' quantitative analysis, has replaced the opinion and belief of experts (Jasper and Rolfe 2011). New governance rules have been established aimed at improving quality through the adoption of business principles and quality indicator reporting. This has

[4] Discussed in Chap. 5.

[5] Discussed in Chap. 3.

[6] Discussed in Chap. 6.

led to an increase in the administrative work of healthcare, with minimal improvement on population health parameters for chronic illness (Anderson 2013).

In summary, built on the principles of Cartesian science, health and healthcare has operated in a paradigm of separation of professions and sub-professions, of patients and professionals and of hierarchies of control. Practices and processes that assume a linear cause and effect association have led to technical (medical) solutions being presaged over patient expertise, with quality performance governed by quantitative measures of performance. This led Noyes (2021) to claim that healthcare is being fueled by the biomedical model in which pharmaceutical companies have significant commercial stakes. Speaking of the impact of mechanization on leadership, Grint (1997, p.10) described this as:

> … rooted in Aristotelian binary logic, where the world is divided into good and bad, right and wrong, truth and lies, black and white, life and death, 0 and 1 and so on. This principle…has encouraged us to perceive our world, and our place in it, as one where clarity of decision-making is premised upon clarity of our perspective.

2.2 A New Paradigm of a Holistic Ecosystem of Health and Healthcare

2.2.1 Principles and Purposes (P1)

As the twentieth century progressed, a new principle of 'body' slowly emerged from the amalgamation of existentialism (Sartre 1957; Camus 1958) and anthropology (Jaspers 1931). Gold (1985, p. 664) described this as envisaging human bodies as "multiphasic, experiential beings of finite freedom." This emergence has been accompanied by an expanded purpose for health and healthcare from disease prevention to treament (Kurdack 2016) based in a 'lived' body, holistic-biopsychological model. Further understanding of the complex world in which health and healthcare operate, together with identification of an array of challenges, has led to recognition of the need to adapt to "ever emergent and concerted or intentional change … in which it is impossible to impose order" (Khan et al. 2018, p. 3). Emerging from this understanding, Complexity science views the word as essentially interconnected, rich with forms and patterns and in a continual process of becoming (Boulton et al. 2015). In this world, complexity thinking requires:

> new perspectives to reassess both natural and human systems…Concepts such as chaos, self organization, dissipative structures and complex adaptive systems began to be used in order to understand both irregular aspects nature displays as well as providing frameworks to explore regularities that arise in complex system. (McDaniel et al. 2013, p. 6)

This understanding has led to claims that health and healthcare need to acknowledge the multilayered and multifaceted contributions required to "open new avenues for understanding the deeply social and discursive nature of complex organisations" (Mannion and Davies 2018, p. 4). Complexity science is based in a holistic philosophy of health and healthcare. New fields of study in health have emerged that are extending consideration of what affects health. This includes occupational and environmental health, the political ecology of health, environmental justice, ecohealth, one health, and ecological public health and planetary health that link health and healthcare to the environment (Buse et al. 2018). While these emergent fields have adopted different approaches and foci, they share a common theme of "explicit recognition of the complex interdependencies among the health of ecosystems, human and other species" (Buse et al. 2018, p. 422). It has also led to discourse about the need for health and healthcare to adopt a more humanistic approach that asks questions to determine what social values are being served by technical solution. This includes questions of what role government should play in the delivery of health services (Schein 1996) and what approaches to the work of healthcare are best designed to promote humanism and practice structures (Rider et al. 2018).

2.2.2 *People in Place (P2)*

Accompanying the call for a more holistic approach to health and healthcare has been discourse on the need to replace the separation of disciplines and professions with more relational approaches that recognize interconnections and integration between parts (Holtman 2011). Building from the research of Dunn and Cummins (2007), Castellani et al. (2015, p. 1) identified the need to recognise the place in which healthcare occurs as:

> integrated; related, places need to be thought of in holistic or systems terms as complex, emergent entities; furthermore, places need to be seen as functioning at multiple levels of scale; operating with open-ended boundaries; fluid, mobile and evolving; not constrained by traditional notions of space and time; comprised of nonlinear feedback loops and causal pathways; with subjective histories and multiple social meanings; emerging out of the intersection of the micro and macro, the local and global, and agency and structure; and, finally, as nodes in a larger network of places and environmental forces. In short, places need to be treated as complex systems.

Bridges et al. (2011, p. 1) highlighted the need for holistic healthcare to champion "more than one discipline ..(*to*).. address issues regarding their health status." In supporting the inclusion of allied health in a holistic approach, Anderson (2013, p. 28) stated that the "intractable problems in health care, because of their complexity, require interprofessional teams to bring various disciplinary perspectives to problem solving, followed by highly coordinated work efforts and effective interdependencies." This requires interactions among interdisciplinary teams to use "real-time information and explore multiple perspectives … to quickly create new knowledge and facilitate the staff's ability to create solutions to emerging problems" (Anderson 2013, p. 30). It led Hartviksen et al. (2018) to claim that good quality care depends upon professions working together in interprofessional teams, with processes and clinical pathways that integrate evidence-based medicine and a focus on treating persons, not diseases, body parts, or organs. Such claims challenge the traditional separation of professions to allow different professions to learn from each other from "an insider's perspective, discovering in that process even other occupational cultures that affect how organizations work" (Schein 1996, p. 239).

Holistic health and healthcare acknowledges that "patients, clients and service users frequently have conditions that have multiple causes and require multiple treatments from a range of health and social care professions with different skills and expertise" (Reeves et al. 2011. p. 13). It highlights the need for co-creation to enable all participants in the delivery of healthcare—patients, administrators and management leaders, physicians and other healthcare professionals, staff and other stakeholders—to reach consensus on the organizational mission, strategy, and goals and through this to develop a shared common vision (Rider et al. 2018). It questions the traditional separation of patients to be replaced by a person-centered approach. Balint (1969), an early supporter of patient-centered medicine, emphasised the need to treat each patient as a unique human being and to increase the 'patient voice' at both the individual and collective level.

Despite these discussions, and some isolated changes, as will be shown more clearly in following chapters, a holistic approach is more rhetoric that reality that requires a more concerted approach to change that links human modes of cognition to understanding of the spiritual, actions to build relationships, and leadership to develop collaboration.

2.2.3 *Practices and Processes (P3)*

What is also under discussion is the change in focus from the individual to a public health purpose. This is demonstrated in primary healthcare (PHC), viewed as a whole—of—society approach. PHC is underpinned by commitment to a more humanistic focus based in a new culture of respect, trust, collaboration, and compassion. PHC consists of three components: (i) integrating health services to meet people's health needs throughout their lives, (ii) addressing the broader determinants of health through multisectoral policy and action, and (iii) empowering individuals, families, and communities to take charge of their own health (WHO https://www.who.int/health-topics/primary-health-care#tab=tab_1). To achieve these aims at the macro level requires change in the design of practices and processes for the delivery of healthcare at the micro level. There is need to design healthcare provision based on the assumption of sequential and simultaneous events (rather than single linear cause and effect relationships) caused by many interdependent components of a system in which output becomes disproportional to the input. Schein (1996, p. 232) described this as planning for "breakthrough research…driven in part by the need to contribute to the solution of highly visible problems." Thygeson et al. (2010) added the need to consider changes to decision-making and leadership, away from individuals in positions of power to regarding leadership as an activity that engages many experts, healthcare managers, and professionals at any level, coproducing care with patients. Mannion and Davies (2018) discussed the need for leadership able to balance different cultures to achieve congruence and complementarity between different cultures, systems, policies, and accountabilities. Others have discussed the need for new approaches, such as distributed leadership to share decision making (Currie and Lockett 2011; Dickson and Tholl 2014; Sebastian et al. 2014), to promote collaboration.

2.3 Discussion

The degree of change required for health and healthcare to adopt a new paradigm is significant. The proposal presented in this book is for a re-imagined paradigm of a holistic ecosystem based in collaboration between three agencies of health and healthcare: Principles and Processes (P1); People in Place (P2); and Practices and Processes (P3).

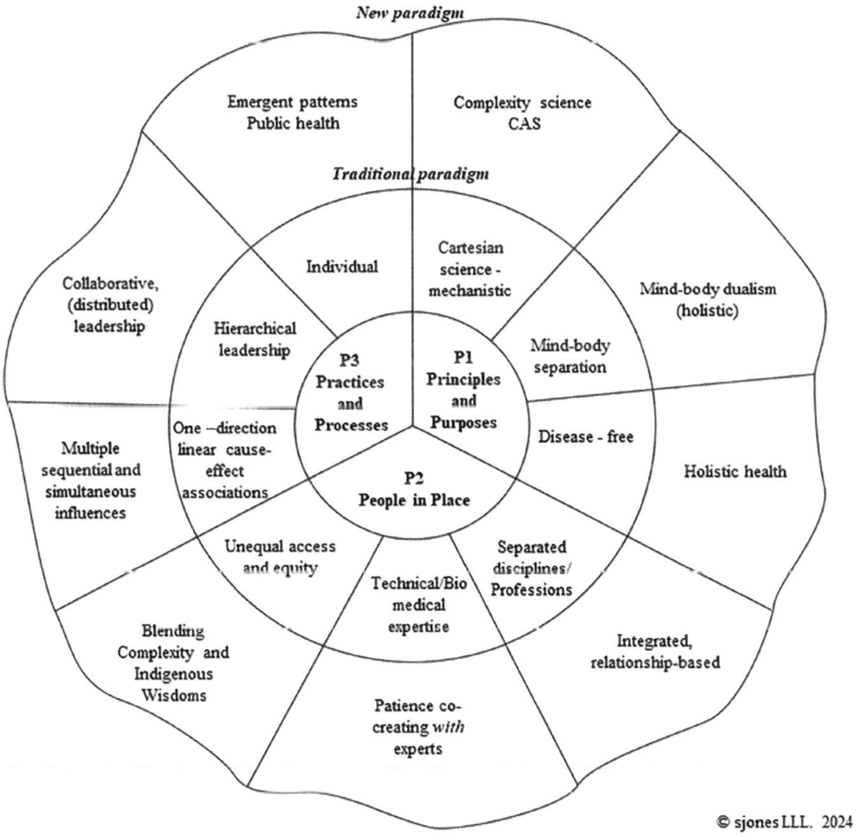

Fig. 2.1 A Holistic Ecosystem of Health and Healthcare: Conjoining Cartesian and Complexity Sciences

This is illustrated in Fig. 2.1 as the three agencies in the inner circle of three inter-related circles. The surrounding circle identifies the principles and practices arising from Cartesian science (termed traditional paradigm). The outer circle identifies the principles and practices arising from Complexity science (termed new paradigm). This depiction allows for consideration of a potential conjoining of principles to transition from the old to the new paradigm to suit different different contexts and cultures. The thinking and action changes that need to be considered to realize health and healthcare as a holistic ecosystem are discussed in chapters in Part II.

2.4 Conclusion

The aim of this chapter was to provide an overview of the changes required in health and healthcare to respond to the complex world. The proposal in this book is for a re-imagined paradigm of health and healthcare as a holistic ecosystem grounded in three agencies of health and healthcare: Principles and Purposes (P1); People in Place (P2); Practices and Processes (P3). The form and extent of change proposed by this paradigm has implications for the way the agencies act and interact. These issues are explored throughout this book.

2.5 Reflective Pause Point

1. Does your experience of health and healthcare, either as a professional or as a patient, accord more closely with what has been described as the traditional paradigm based in Cartesian science or an emergent paradigm based in Complexity science?
2. Reflecting on your experiences, how might adoption of one element (choose any one) of the emergent paradigm contribute to an improved quality of health and healthcare?
3. Of the three agencies of health and healthcare identified, which do you consider you may have most opportunity to change?

References

Anderson R (2013) Commentary on health care organizations as complex systems: new perspectives on design and management. Adv Health Care Manag 15:27–36

Balint E (1969) The possibilities of patient-centered medicine. J R Coll Gen Pract 17(82):269–276

Boulton JG, Allen PM, Bowman C (2015) Embracing complexity: strategic perspectives for an age of turbulence. Oxford University Press

Bridges D, Davidson A, Soule Odegard P et al (2011) Interprofessional collaboration: three best practice models of interprofessional education. Medical Education Online Trend Article
Buse CG, Oestreicher JS, Ellis NR et al (2018) Public health guide to field developments linking ecosystems, environments and health in the Anthropocene. J Epidemiol Community Health 72:420–425
Camus A (1958) L'Envers et l'Endroit. Gatlimard, Paris. In: Lyrical-Critical Essays. Vintage Books, (1970), New York
Castellani B, Rjaram R, Buckwalter JG et al (2015) Place and health as complex systems: a case-study and empirical test, Springer Briefs in Public Health. Springer. https://doi.org/10.1007/978-3-319-09734-3
Currie G, Lockett A (2011) Distributed leadership in health and social care: concertive, conjoint or collective. Int J Manag Rev 13:286–300. https://doi.org/10.1111/j.1468-2370.2011.00308.x
Dickson G, Tholl B (2014) Bringing leadership to life in health: LEADS in a caring environment a new perspective. Springer-Verlag, London
Dunn J, Cummins S (2007) Placing health in context [editorial]. Soc Sci Med 65:1821–1824
Gislason M, Bendelow G (2013) Introduction. In: Gislason M (ed) Ecological health: society. Ecology and Health, Emerald Publishing Limited
Gold J (1985) Cartesian dualism and the current crisis in medicine – a plea for a philosophical approach; discussion paper. J R Soc Med 78:663–666
Grint K (1997) Leadership: classical, contemporary, and critical approaches. University Press, Oxford
Hart N (1985) The sociology of health and medicine. Causeway Press, Lancashire
Hartviksen T, Sjolie B, Aspfors J et al (2018) Healthcare middle managers experiences developing leadership capacity and capability in a public funded learning network. BMC Health Sci Res 18:433. https://doi.org/10.1186/s12913-018-3259-
Holtman M (2011) Paradoxes of professionalism and error in complex systems. J Biomed Inform 44:395–401
Jasper M, Rolfe G (2011) The emergence of professional knowledge. In: Rolfe G, Jasper M, Freshwater D (eds) Critical reflection in practice, Ch 2. Palgrave Macmillan, Basingstoke, Hampshire, pp 11–29
Jaspers K (1931) Die Geistige der Zeit (Man in the Modem Age). RKP, (1951), London
Khan S, Vandermorris A, Shepherd J et al (2018) Embracing uncertainty, managing complexity: applying complexity thinking principles to transformation efforts in healthcare systems. BMC Health Serv Res 18:192. https://doi.org/10.1186/s12913-018-2994-
Kurdack H (2016) Finding wholeness: which research method can be useful in putting together the puzzle in medicine divided into pieces by Cartesian philosophy? JSM Health Educ Prim Health Care 1(2):1016
Mannion R, Davies H (2018) Understanding organisational culture for healthcare quality improvement. BMJ Open Access 363:k4907. https://doi.org/10.1136/bmj.k4907
McDaniel RR Jr, Driebe DJ, Lanham HJ (2013) Health care organizations as complex systems: new perspectives on design and management. Adv Health Care Manag 15:3–26. https://doi.org/10.1108/s1474-8231(2013)0000015007. PMID: 24749211.
Mehta N (2011) Mind-body dualism: a critique from a health perspective. In: Singh AR, Singh SA (eds) Brain, mind & consciousness: An international, interdisciplinary perspective. MSM, 9(1):202–209
Noyes A (2021) Navigating the hierarchy: communicating power relationships in collaborative health care groups. Manag Commun Q 36(1):62–91
Parmelli E, Flodgren G, Beyer F et al (2011) The effectiveness of strategies to change organisational culture to improve healthcare performance: a systematic review. Implement Sci 6(33). https://doi.org/10.1186/1748-5908-6-33
Pomey M-P, Ghadiri DP, Karazivan P et al (2015) Patients as partners: a qualitative study of patients' engagement in their health care. PLoS One 10(4):e0122499. https://doi.org/10.1371/journal.pone.0122499

Reeves S, Zwarenstein M, Espin S et al (2011) Interprofessional teamwork for health and social care. John Wiley & Sons

Rider EA, Gilligan MC, Osterberg LG et al (2018) Healthcare at the crossroads: the need to shape an organizational culture of humanistic teaching and practice. J Gen Intern Med 33:1092–1099

Sartre J-P (1957) L'Ttre et le Neant. Gallimard, Paris. In: Being and nothingness. Translator H

Schein E (1996) Culture: the missing concept in organizations studies. Adm Sci Q 41:229–240

Sebastian A, Fulop L, Dadich A et al (2014) Health LEADS Australia and implications for medical leadership. Leadersh Health Serv 27(4):355–370

Thygeson M, Morrissey L, Ulstad V. (2010) Adaptive leadership and the practice of medicine: a complexity-based approach to reframing the doctor-patient relationship. Journal of Evaluative Clinical Practice. 16(5):1009–15.

Thygeson M (2013) Implementing adaptive health practice: a complexity-based philosophy of health care. In: Sturmberg JP, Martin CM (eds) Handbook of systems and complexity in health. Springer Science + Business, Media, NY, pp 661–684. https://doi.org/10.1007/978-1-4614-4998-0_38

Tuffin R (2016) Implications of complexity theory for clinical practice and healthcare organization. Br J Anaesth 16(10):349–352

World Health Organization (WHO) (1946) Preamble to the Constitution of the World Health Organization as adopted by the International Health Conference, 19–22

Chapter 3
Impact of Cartesian Science on Indigenous Health

Dein Vindigni OAM, Uncle Paul Callaghan, and Uncle Paul Gordon

Abstract This chapter presents an overview of the impact of Cartesian science, and the mechanistic thinking that has accompanied it, on the health of Indigenous people. The chapter identifies the challenges faced by Indigenous people in many countries that has resulted from the clash of philosophies as Western countries, influenced by Cartesian science, have sought to colonize Indigenous people. These challenges to traditional Indigenous values and Indigenous ways of life and the separation of Indigenous people from country have led to an ever-escalating negative impact on Indigenous health and well-being.

3.1 Introduction

Indigenous peoples belong to the longest continuous cultures on Earth (Chandler and Lalonde 1998; Goodes et al. 2021). The meaning of the term "Indigenous" varies among anthropologists and even among Indigenous people themselves (Kuper 2005, p. 983). It is used in some settings to include the Aboriginal population of a nation or the first recorded inhabitants of that nation. In Australia, it includes the Aboriginal and Torres Strait Islander peoples of Australia, although even this generic term is not recognized by many Aboriginal 'mobs' that are grouped under this banner. In New Zealand, it relates to the Māori people; in Canada to the Inuit, Metis, Cree, and Dene peoples; and in Latin America to the Guarani, May, Yanomami, and Aymara peoples (Anderson et al. 2006; Montenegro and Stephens 2006; Sylvain 2002). In other countries, the term "Indigenous" is used to refer to groups of people who claim indigeneity compared with white

D. Vindigni OAM (✉)
STEM College, RMIT University, Melbourne, VIC, Australia
e-mail: dein.vindigni@rmit.edu.au

U. P. Callaghan · U. P. Gordon
University of New England, Armidale, NSW, Australia

S. Jones, D. Vindigni OAM (eds.), *Health and Healthcare in Complexity*,
https://doi.org/10.1007/978-981-96-0515-6_3

colonists, such as the black Africans in Africa (Sylvain 2002). In yet other countries, it is used to refer to groups of people living in communities, such as the Adivasi people in India, who live in tribal, forest communities and have a distinct language and cultural practices aligned with nature (Government of India 1949). According to Sepie (2017), the root definition of Indigenous is 'people springing from/in the land as mother.'

In the 1990s, the World Bank (1993) adopted the criterion of "self-identification as Indigenous," coupled with being accepted by Indigenous people as part of that community. As the challenges and negative impacts of climate change have become more visible, many Indigenous people are reclaiming the land, lore, kinship, and language from which they were historically disconnected (Rose 1999; Kelly et al. 2012). This has also resulted in Indigenous peoples proudly reclaiming their heritage.

While recognizing that self-identification has been contested by members of some Indigenous communities, it does provide a basis upon which to gather data about Indigenous people. Bell (2014, p. 83) stated some members of Indigenous communities either fear they will be "swamped" by "wannabes" or are concerned that self-identification is being used by "modern-day settler-colonialism which seeks to either relegate the indigene to primitivism or assimilate them completely into settler identities." Amnesty International (2023) recently estimated that there are currently over 476 million Indigenous people who represent about 5% of the world's population. Indigenous people live in over 90 countries and belong to more than 5,000 different peoples, speaking more than 5,000 languages. In Australia, for example, Karulkiyalu Country, Gordon and Spillman (2021, p.216) stated that "it is estimated that in 1788 when the British stepped onto the Australian shore now known as Sydney, there were up to 600 different language groups across Australia, all composed of various clans, tribal or familial groups, each responsible for their Country." Despite these numbers and geographic spread, most Indigenous peoples coexist in modern socioeconomic and political contexts with non-Indigenous people, although many continue to embrace a connection with, and reverence for, nature (McGregor 2020).

3.2 Indigenous Health

The health of Indigenous peoples is affected by different challenges than those confronting non-Indigenous peoples. Despite the wealth of their traditional knowledges and wisdom, Indigenous people continue to be among the poorest and most marginalized throughout the world and experience poorer health than non-Indigenous people living in the same countries (Stephens et al. 2005; Anderson et al. 2006; Montenegro and Stephens 2006; Sylvain 2002; Di 2016; Carson et al. 2020). Although the accuracy of information relating to the health status of Indigenous people throughout the world varies considerably (Coimbra et al. 2004; Fremantle et al. 2008), it is acknowledged that they suffer a wider range and burden of illnesses than those experienced by non-Indigenous people (Valeggia and Snodgrass 2015). Indigenous peoples have a higher incidence of most diseases, including diabetes, cardiovascular disease, mental illness, and cancers (Deravin et al. 2018), and generally a lower life expectancy than non-Indigenous people (King et al. 2009; Gracey and King 2009; Zhao et al. 2013; Tjepkema et al. 2019). A common finding across all Indigenous communities is higher rates of infant mortality (Chen et al. 2015; Freemantle et al. 2006; Black et al. 2003; Lawn et al. 2005; Victoria et al. 2003; Rudan et al. 2005).

In Australia, for example, statistics show that Indigenous people comprise approximately 3.3% of the total Australian population (about 800,000 out of 24 million people) (Australian Bureau of Statistics 2018). Indigenous Australians are recognized as consisting of two distinct cultural groups—the Aboriginal people and the Torres Strait Islander people—who traditionally speak over 250 distinct languages across the nation (AIATSIS 2018), although they are collectively identified as Aboriginal and Torres Strait Islander people. However, it is also acknowledged that Indigenous Australians experience widespread socioeconomic disadvantage and health inequality (Australian Institute of Health and Welfare 2017). The most recent national survey by the Australian Bureau of Statistics (ABS 2019) identified Aboriginal and Torres Strait Islander people as having a higher level of disease (2.3 times that of non-Indigenous Australians), higher rates of psychological distress, and a range of chronic health conditions. For example, 46% of Aboriginal and Torres Strait Islander people have at least one chronic condition: 10.7% with asthma, 1.5% with chronic obstructive pulmonary disease, 5.3% with diabetes, 4% with heart disease, 1.1% with kidney disease, 20.1% with mental or behavioral conditions, 31% with psychological distress, and 14% with ear disease or a hearing problem (HealthInfoNet AI et al. 2018). In their recent book on Australian Indigenous peoples, Callaghan and Gordon (2023) referred to poor health status of Indigenous Australians, including higher death rates (1.8x), more preventable hospitalizations (2.9x), greater levels of cardiovascular disease (1.2x), higher rates of cancer (1.1x), increased incidents of diabetes (3.5x), higher levels of psychological distress (2.7x), greater levels of kidney disease (6.8x), higher rates of injury (1.2x), higher rates of respiratory illness (1.2x), and higher levels of eye-health problems (3x). These higher rates of poor health are attributed to a range of factors varying from poor environmental health, nutrition and breastfeeding, physical activity, bodyweight, immunization, alcohol use, illicit drug use, and volatile-substance use. Although there is some evidence that the life expectancy for Indigenous Australians is improving, it is recognized that the closing of this gap is unacceptably slow (Ring and Griffiths 2022).

3.3 Causes of Poor Indigenous Health: Colonization

While the causes of Indigenous people's poor health are many, complex, and varied (Stephens et al. 2006), social and cultural marginalization has been reported as a key determinant (King et al. 2009; Crocetti et al. 2022). It is further recognized that social and cultural marginalization has itself resulted from historical, social, economic, and cultural impacts of British colonization on settler colonies in Australia, the USA, Canada, and New Zealand (Smith 2005; Archibald 2006). These British settlers bought with them the mechanistic thinking that grew from Cartesian science that clashed with traditional Indigenous values and Indigenous ways of life. It separated Indigenous people from country and from the ancient wisdoms upon which their culture and their commune with nature, and with each other, were built. The impact of this clash of philosophies has been negative, on Indigenous ways of knowing, being, and doing, and on Indigenous health and well-being. In each of the cases highlighted in this chapter, colonization has led to the loss of culture, language, land, and resources and progressive environmental degradation and sociocultural dispossession, as well as the denial of political, religious, and personal freedoms and the misappropriation of lands from Indigenous people (Kiddle 2020; Axelsson et al. 2016). The misappropriation of land, the displacement and eradication of communities through genocide, the introduction of diseases, enforcement of policies of assimilation, institutionalization of systemic racism, and discrimination are described by Paradies (2016, p. 88) as:

> notably, colonisation and racism are concepts often paired in discourse, with an implicit assumption that colonisation temporally precedes and has 'caused' racism against Indigenous peoples, while the salience of racism now outlives the more historically-inflected phenomenon of colonisation.

Leading climate scientists have acknowledged that colonization is a historic and ongoing driver of the climate crisis and adversely affects world populations in general as well as the health and well-being of Indigenous people who are the traditional custodians of the colonized lands (Evolve Communities 2024). Paradies (2016, pp. 83–84) described colonization as encompassing a range of historical practices that may include "war, displacement, forced labour, removal of children, relocation, ecological destruction, genocide, slavery, (un)intentional spread of deadly diseases, banning of Indigenous languages, regulation of marriage, assimilation and eradication of social, cultural and spiritual practices." While recognizing that colonization is not exclusive to Indigenous people, Paradies (2016) explained that what makes the domination of a settler majority group distinct for Indigenous people is the status that the first peoples lost. For Indigenous Australian peoples, British colonization resulted in dispossession, physical ill-treatment, social disruption, population decline, economic exploitation, codified discrimination, and cultural devastation (Czyzewski 2011; Ramos 2020).[1]

These losses have been associated with the persistent poor health and lower social and economic status of Indigenous people (Smith 2005; Archibald 2006). Many lives were lost due to the proliferation of epidemics such as measles and smallpox (Valeggia and Snodgrass 2015, Evolve Communities 2024). Health inequities continue to be widespread among Indigenous populations, underpinned by social and cultural determinants of Indigenous health and well-being (Curtis et al. 2019; Atkinson 2002; Czyzewski 2011; Ramos 2020). For Indigenous Australians, the long-term impact has been compounded by intergenerational and

[1] For details of the chronology, see Callaghan and Gordon 2023.

transgenerational trauma (Hollinsworth 2010; Hinton et al. 2014). Zubrick et al. (2004, p. 99) stated:

> Many of the unique risks faced by Aboriginal peoples have persisted across generations. This reflects the fact that the health and wellbeing of Aboriginal peoples has been profoundly shaped by the circumstances of the past, and most particularly by the events and conditions in Australia since colonisation. The enduring legacy of colonisation on Aboriginal life has been pervasive and affected multiple generations and extends to all dimensions of the holistic notion of Aboriginal wellbeing, including psychological, social, spiritual and cultural aspects of life and connection to land. This has resulted in serious additional risks to wellbeing, including: unresolved grief and loss; trauma and abuse; violence; removal from family; substance misuse; family breakdown; cultural dislocation; racism and discrimination; exclusion and segregation; loss of control of life; and social disadvantage.

Uncle Paul Gordon (an Australian Aboriginal Elder) paints a poignant picture:

> Imagine a world where people have all they need to be contented. Where they live to be old and are happy in mind, body, and spirit. That is the way our people lived for a very, very long time. Life could sometimes be hard, but our knowledge of the land meant that we always had what we needed. (Callaghan with Gordon 2023, p. 22)

This situation changed with the British colonization in the late 1700s. This was described by Uncle Paul Gordon (Vindigni 2004, p.12):

> At the end of the 19th century, Queen Victoria ordered the creation of missions to protect Aboriginal people from being shot by early settlers. Aboriginal people were regularly rounded up from nearby and even distant communities to the missions. From these original benevolent intentions, the efforts to 'civilise' Aboriginal people soon saw them prevented from hunting, gathering, eating their nutritious bush foods and using bush medicines to promote their health and wellbeing. They were forced to live on the mission and survive on rations of sugar, tea, coffee and refined flour. This diet and its legacy of poor health continues to affect Aboriginal people today. They were forbidden to speak their language, practise their spiritual beliefs or hunt and gather foods. Working for white farmers became their principal occupation. This involved shearing sheep, droving cattle, fencing and picking cotton.

Australians together (2019) have described the consequences of these changes:

> Land, family, law, ceremony, and language are five key interconnected elements of Indigenous culture…the five elements combine to create a way of seeing and being in the world that is distinctly Indigenous. Understanding how intricately interconnected these elements are, helps us understand the damage done when colonisation occurred. Being disconnected from culture can have a profound impact on a person's sense of identity and belonging. Identity and belonging give meaning and purpose to people's lives. Understanding this will help us find appropriate ways to respond to the pain caused by colonisation.

Similarly, Atkinson (2002, p. 71) wrote about 'cultural genocide,' which:

> not only works to destroy the cultures of oppressed peoples, it also eradicates the sense of self, of self-worth and of wellbeing in individuals and groups so that they are unable to function from either their own cultural relatedness, or from the culture of the oppressors. They feel in a world between, devalued, and devaluing who they are.

This has resulted in Indigenous Australians remaining the most disadvantaged and marginalized group in Australia:

> Colonisation has left a devastating impact on Aboriginal and Torres Strait Islander communities and culture…. Indigenous Australians have suffered ongoing inter-generational trauma. These factors are recognised as having a fundamental impact on the disadvantage and poor physical and mental health of Indigenous peoples worldwide…. In contrast, Aboriginal and Torres Strait Islander cultural identity and participation in cultural activities…are recognised as protective factors and can positively influence overall health and wellbeing. (Australian Institute of Health and Welfare 2022)

In the words of Uncle Paul Gordon,[2] the outcome has been despair for young Aboriginal (Indigenous) people who are scarred by their knowledge of the loss of their culture, their land, and their hope:

> Seeing the land bulldozed for farming or dug up for mining is like a non-Aboriginal person returning to their home to find their own mother lying on the floor, bleeding. The feeling of hurt and of horror is the same in both cases.

The negative impact is also highlighted by Uncle Bob Randall (an Elder of the Yankunytjatjara people from Central Australia), in his film Kanyini (2006) (https://www.kanyini.com/), in which he highlights the importance of culture and ancient wisdom in achieving a state of well-being for Indigenous Australians. Uncle Bob explains the term 'kanyini' as a sacred principle of responsibility and unconditional love for all of creation. Using his language, the four main areas of responsibility he cites are tjukurrpa (philosophy, law, and religion), ngura (home and country), waltyja (family and kinship), and kurunpa (spirit, soul, and psyche). In a particularly powerful and emotive part of the film, he reinforces the impacts of colonization and cultural genocide when he states "You take away my kanyini, my connectedness, I'm nothing, I'm dead, I'm a corpse in space."

In summary, negative health impacts for Indigenous peoples have resulted from colonization, the associated policies to assimilate and acculturate Indigenous peoples into the ways of the dominant colonial power, and the marginalization and alienation they have experienced. This is poignantly captured in the words of an Australian Indigenous media personality, Stan Grant (Ethics Centre 2016):

> We heard a howl. We heard a howl of humiliation that echoes across two centuries of dispossession, injustice, suffering and survival. We heard the howl of the Australian dream and it said to us again, you are not welcome. The Australian Dream. We sing of it, and we recite it in verse. Australians all, let us rejoice for we are young and free. My people die young in this country. We die ten years younger than average Australians and we are far from free.

3.4 Where to from Here?

Before Indigenous peoples can experience a better health future, there is need for a paradigm shift in thinking that recognizes the importance of a deep personal sense of meaning and purpose as indispensable to one's health and well-being. This requires recognition of culture, that is, "the spiritual, emotional, and social growth and

[2] Coauthor of this chapter.

maintenance of all peoples…culture is their spear and shield; their resistance and their resilience" (Frankland et al. 2011, p. 27). All people need to feel that their sense of self and identity is valued and appreciated by the people and environments that comprise their lives and that beyond any differences they feel respected and culturally safe (Bouma et al. 2011). It also requires a focus on personalized medicine (Lippi and Plebani 2015) that tailors the medical model more closely to the individual. This is explained by the European Union Council (2015, p. 3) as the need for:

> a medical model using characterisation of individuals' phenotypes and genotypes (e.g. molecular profiling, medical imaging, lifestyle data) for tailoring the right therapeutic strategy for the right person at the right time, and/or to determine the predisposition to disease and/or to deliver timely and targeted prevention.

3.5 Conclusion

This chapter has presented an overview of the negative impact of colonization by Western countries, influenced by Cartesian science, on the health of Indigenous peoples. The poor health of Indigenous peoples in countries colonized by Western powers is attributed to the disconnection of Indigenous people from their ancestral lands and lore which has led to a loss of culture and identity. This provides context for a later discussion in Part II (Chaps. 11 and 12) which identifies how a strength-based approach anchored in Ancient Indigenous Wisdoms, culture, and connection to country, is the first step toward improving Indigenous health.

References

Amnesty International (2023). Available at: https://www.amnesty.org/en/what-we-do/indigenous-peoples/#:~:text=Overview,5%25%20of%20the%20world's%20population

Anderson I, Crengle S, Kamaka ML, Chen TH, Palafox N, Jackson-Pulver L (2006) Indigenous health in Australia, New Zealand, and the Pacific. Lancet 367(9524):1775–1785

Archibald L (2006) Decolonization and healing: indigenous experiences in the United States, New Zealand, Australia and Greenland. Aboriginal Healing Foundation, Ottawa

Atkinson J (2002) Trauma trails, recreating song lines: the transgenerational effects of trauma in Indigenous Australia. Spinifex Press

Australian Bureau of Statistics (2018) Estimates of Aboriginal and Torres Strait Islander Australians – June 2016. (Catalogue No. 3238.0.55.001). Retrieved from https://www.abs.gov.au/ausstats/abs@.nsf/mf/3238.0.55.001

Australian Bureau of Statistics (2019) National Aboriginal and Torres Strait Islander Health Survey. Viewed 11 January 2023, https://www.abs.gov.au/statistics/people/aboriginal-and-torres-strait-islander-peoples/national-aboriginal-and-torres-strait-islander-health-survey/latest-release

Australian Institute of Aboriginal and Torres Strait Islander Studies [AIATSIS] (2018) Indigenous Australians: Aboriginal and Torres Strait Islander people. Retrieved from https://aiatsis.gov.au/explore/articles/indigenous-australians-aboriginal-and-torres-strait-islander-people

Australian Institute of Health and Welfare (2017) Australia's Welfare 2017: In brief Australian Institute of Health and Welfare. Viewed 4 January 2023, https://www.aihw.gov.au/reports/australias-welfare/australias-welfare-2017-in-brief/contents/indigenous-australians

Australian Institute of Health and Welfare (2022) Determinants of health for Indigenous Australians, Australian Institute of Health and Welfare. Viewed 4 January 2023, https://www.aihw.gov.au/reports/australias-health/social-determinants-and-indigenous-health

Australians Together (2019) Why are culture and identity important? Australians Together, viewed 10 March 2020. Viewed https://australianstogether.org.au/discover/indigenous-culture/culture-identity/

Axelsson P, Kukutai T, Kippen R (2016) The field of Indigenous health and the role of colonisation and history. J Popul Res 33:1–7

Bell A (2014) Relating indigenous and settler identities: beyond domination. Palgrave Macmillan, New York

Black RE, Morris SS, Bryce J (2003) Where and why are 10 million children dying every year? Lancet 361:2226–2234

Bouma G, Cahill D, Dellal H, Zwartz A (2011) Freedom of religion and belief in 21st century Australia: a research report prepared for the Australian human rights commission. Australian Human Rights Commission

Callaghan P with Uncle Paul Gordon (2023) The dreaming path: Indigenous thinking to change your life. HarperONE isbn-13 978-0063321267

Carson B, Dunbar T, Chenhall RD, Bailie R (eds) (2020) Social determinants of indigenous health. Routledge

Chandler MJ, Lalonde C (1998) Cultural continuity as a hedge against suicide in Canada's first nations. Transcult Psychiatry 35(2):191–219

Chen L, Xiao L, Auger N, Torrie J, McHugh NGL, Zoungrana H, Luo ZC (2015) Disparities and trends in birth outcomes, perinatal and infant mortality in Aboriginal vs. non-Aboriginal populations: a population-based study in Quebec, Canada 1996–2010. PLoS One 10(9):e0138562

Coimbra CE, Santos RV, Salzano FM, Hurtado AM (2004) Emerging health needs and epidemiologic research in indigenous peoples in Brazil. In: Salzano FM, Hurtado M (eds) Lost paradise and the ethics of research and publication. Oxford University Press, Oxford, pp 89–109

Crocetti AC, Cubillo B, Lock M, Walker T, Hill K, Mitchell F, Paradies Y, Backholer K, Browne J (2022) The commercial determinants of indigenous health and well-being: a systematic scoping review. BMJ Glob Health 7(11):e010366

Curtis E, Jones R, Tipene-Leach D, Walker C, Loring B, Paine SJ, Reid P (2019) Why cultural safety rather than cultural competency is required to achieve health equity: a literature review and recommended definition. Int J Equity Health 18(1):1–17

Czyzewski K (2011) Colonialism as a broader social determinant of health. Int Indig Policy J 2(1)

Deravin L, Francis K, Anderson J (2018) Closing the gap in indigenous health inequity–is it making a difference? Int Nurs Rev 65(4):477–483

Di A (2016) Indigenous health: a worldwide focus. Cancer 755(45358):576325

Ethics Centre (2016) Stan Grant: racism and the Australian dream, Ethics Centre. Viewed on 11 January 2023. https://ethics.org.au/stan-grants-speech/

European Union (2015) Council conclusion on personalised medicine for patients. Off J Eur Union C421

Evolve communities, http://www.evolves.com.a

Frankland R, Bamblett M, Lewis P (2011) 'Forever business': a framework for maintaining and restoring cultural safety in Aboriginal Victoria [online]. Indigenous Law Bulletin 7(24):27–30. May/June Retrieved from https://search.informit.com.au/documentSummary;dn=2112559235493 58;res=IELAPA. ISSN: 1328-5475

Fremantle CJ, Read AW, de Klerk NH, McAullay D, Anderson IP, Stanley FJ (2006) Patterns, trends, and increasing disparities in mortality for aboriginal and non-aboriginal infants born in Western Australia, 1980–2001: population database study. Lancet 367(9524):758–1766

Fremantle E, Zurynski YA, Mahajan D, D'Antoine H, Elliott EJ (2008) Indigenous child health: urgent need for improved data to underpin better health outcomes. Med J Aust 188(10):588–591

Goodes A, Laing E, Hardy D (2021) Somebody's land. Allen & Unwin, Sydney

Government of India (1949) The Constitution of India. Government of India, New Delhi

Gracey M, King M (2009) Indigenous health part 1: determinants and disease patterns. Lancet 374(9683):65–75

HealthInfoNet AI, Harford-Mills M, MacRae A, Drew N (2018) Summary of Aboriginal and Torres Strait Islander health status. Australian Indigenous HealthInfoNet

Hinton AL, Woolford A, Benvenuto J (eds) (2014) Colonial genocide in indigenous North America. Duke University Press

Hollinsworth D (2010) Racism and Indigenous people in Australia. Global Dialogue (Online) 12(2):1

Kanyini (2006). https://www.kanyini.com/. Directed by Melanie Hogan, Mutitjulu, Northern Territory

Karulkiyalu Country, Gordon P, Spillman D (2021) Embracing country as teacher in outdoor and environmental education. In: Thomas G, Dyment J, Prince H (eds) Outdoor environmental education in higher education, (9): 215–224. Springer

Kelly J, Saggers S, Taylor K, Pearce G, Massey P, Bull J, Ahboo S (2012) Makes you proud to be black eh?: reflections on meaningful Indigenous research participation. Int J Equity Health 11:1–8

Kiddle R (2020) Colonisation sucks for everyone. In: Imagining decolonisation. Bridget Williams Books, pp 83–106

King M, Smith A, Gracey M (2009) Indigenous health part 2: the underlying causes of the health gap. Lancet 374(9683):76–85

Kuper A (2005) Indigenous people: an unhealthy category Lancet 366:983

Lawn JE, Cousens S, Zupan J (2005) 4 million neonatal deaths: when? Where? Why? Lancet 365:891–900

Lippi G, Plebani M (2015) Personalized medicine: moving from simple theory to daily practice. CCLM 53(7):959–960

McGregor D (2020) Mother Earth. An insider's guide to a rapidly changing planet. Open Book Publishers, p 133

Montenegro RA, Stephens C (2006) Indigenous health in Latin America and the Caribbean. Lancet 367(9525):1859–1869

Paradies Y (2016) Colonisation, racism and indigenous health. J Popul Res 33(8):3–96

Ramos S (2020) Indigenous apocalypse and transgenerational trauma. AMA J Ethics 22(10):898–903

Ring IT, Griffiths K (2022) Life expectancy for Indigenous people is improving, but closing the gap remains unacceptably slow. Med J Aust 217(1):26–27

Rose DB (1999) Indigenous ecologies and an ethic of connection. In: Low N (ed) Global ethics and environment. Routledge, New York, pp 175–187

Rudan I, Lawn J, Cousens S et al (2005) Gaps in policy-relevant information on burden of disease in children: a systematic review. Lancet 365:2031–2040

Sepie AJ (2017) More than stories, more than myths: animal/ human/nature(s) in traditional ecological worldviews. Humanities 6(78):1–31

Smith TL (2005) On tricky ground: researching the native in the age of uncertainty. In: Denzin N, Lincoln YS (eds) The Sage handbook of qualitative research, 3rd edn. Sage Publications, Thousand Oaks, CA, pp 85–107

Stephens C, Nettleton C, Porter J, Willis R, Clark S (2005) Indigenous peoples' health—why are they behind everyone, everywhere? Lancet 366(9479):10–13

Stephens C, Porter J, Nettleton C, Willis R (2006) Disappearing, displaced, and undervalued: a call to action for Indigenous health worldwide. Lancet 367(9527):2019–2028

Sylvain R (2002) Land, Water and Truth. Am Anthropol 104:1074–1085

Tjepkema M, Bushnik T, Bougie E (2019) Life expectancy of first nations, Métis and Inuit household populations in Canada. Health Rep 30(12):3-10.S
Valeggia CR, Snodgrass JJ (2015) Health of indigenous peoples. Annu Rev Anthropol 44:117–135
Victoria CG, Wagstaff A, Schellenberg JA, Gwatkin D, Claeson M, Habicht JP (2003) Applying an equity lens to child health and mortality: more of the same is not enough. Lancet 362:233–241
Vindigni D (2004). Promoting the musculoskeletal Health of indigenous Australians living in rural communities. Aboriginal Health in Aboriginal communities. Doctoral thesis
World Bank (1993) HRO Dissemination Notes Number 8, Human Resources Development and Operations Policy
Zhao Y, Wright J, Begg S, Guthridge S (2013) Decomposing Indigenous life expectancy gap by risk factors: a life table analysis. Popul Health Metrics 11:1–9
Zubrick S.R, Dudgeon P, Gee, G, et al (2004). Social determinants of Aboriginal and Torres Strait Islander social and emotional wellbeing. Working together, 75.

Chapter 4
Integrating the Professions

Sandra Jones and Dein Vindigni OAM

Abstract The aim of this chapter is to identify changes that have been made to reduce the separation between the healthcare professions and sub professions. The chapter presents two approaches that have been designed to achieve greater integration: interprofessional collaboration and interprofessional education. This discussion is complemented by reflection by the editors to identify the implications for change for each of the 3P agencies of health and healthcare identified in Chapter 1: Principles and Purposes (P1); People in Place (P2); and Practices and Processes (P3).

4.1 Introduction

We saw in Chap. 2 that the World Health Organization (WHO) has urged the adoption of primary healthcare (PHC) to adopt "a whole-of-society approach designed to effectively organize and strengthen national health systems to bring services for health and wellbeing closer to communities" (WHO https://www.who.int/health-topics/primary-health-care#tab=tab_1). PHC outlines a vision for healthcare built on three components: (i) integrating health services to meet people's health needs throughout their lives, (ii) addressing the broader determinants of health through multisectoral policy and action, and (iii) empowering individuals, families, and communities to take charge of their own health. It is to the first of these components, integrating health services, that this chapter is dedicated.

The WHO Operational Framework for PHC (WHO 2020) identified as one of the four key strategic levers, the importance of the "engagement of communities

S. Jones (✉)
Business and Law College, RMIT University, Melbourne, VIC, Australia

D. Vindigni OAM
STEM College, RMIT University, Melbourne, VIC, Australia
e-mail: dein.vindigni@rmit.edu.au

S. Jones, D. Vindigni OAM (eds.), *Health and Healthcare in Complexity*,
https://doi.org/10.1007/978-981-96-0515-6_4

and other stakeholders from all sectors to define problems and solutions and prioritize actions through policy dialogue." It acknowledged that this change is required given the negative impacts of the historic separation of healthcare professions. At the macro level, this has resulted in: the creation of monopolies of power and control based on exclusive knowledge (Illich 1981); the regulation of labor to protect market niches (Witz 1992); and the creation of a system of medicine organized to reflect middle- and upper-class values (Ponte et al. 2003). These criticisms have resulted in healthcare being described as an archetypical bureaucracy "in which a core group of professionals maintain institutional boundaries that can in turn inhibit interprofessional knowledge transfer" (Tasselli 2015, p. 842). At the micro-level, it has led to the development of poor processes and quality of healthcare delivery through, what Hall (2005, p. 190) described as, "conflict and strain between professions", that has resulted in "serious care failures and shortfalls in performance relative to expectations" (Beirne 2017, p. 2). This has led to hierarchical leadership and unequal decision-making that is slanted toward physicians (Lancaster et al. 2015; McKimm 2011; Tasselli 2015), and to "highly complex interrelated relationship-driven characteristics of healthcare organisations" (Hartviksen et al. 2018, p. 2). This has made it difficult to achieve collaboration (D'Amour et al. 2005).

Actions advocated to achieve integration and collaboration in health and healthcare have included the development of "models of care that promote high-quality, people-centred primary care and essential public health functions as the core of integrated health services throughout the course of life" (WHO 2020, p. 4–5). It has led to new models for nursing (Way et al. 2000), mental health and primary care (Kates and Craven 1999). These models have aimed to "more nimbly tackle problems at the interface of human, animal and environmental health" (Steele et al. 2022, p. 4 59). Specific changes implemented under these models have included the encouragement of multispecialty medical groups at the organizational (hospital) level (Burns et al. 2013) and the integration of psychological, social, and medical responses (Silver and Baima 2013).

Despite these attempts to overcome traditional professional separation, there has been limited success. This is due to many factors that range from differences in values, beliefs, attitudes, customs, and behaviors (Schroeder et al. 1999) to the active resistance to transcending hierarchies (Kinnaman and Bleich 2004).

4.2 Interprofessional Collaboration (IPC)

Interprofessional collaboration (IPC) underpins an integrated approach by linking professions working in general practice, community health centers, and allied health clinics (Reddy 2017). IPC has been described as "a type of interprofessional work which involves different health and social care professions who regularly come together to solve problems or provide services" (Reeves et al. 2010, p. 8). IPC acknowledges the "unique expertise of various health and care professions while encouraging them to work together in coordinated care, streamline services and optimise treatment" (Fox and Reeves 2015, p. 113).

Actions taken to promote IPC include the establishment of teams together with encouragement for collaboration, coordination, and networking among professionals (Reeves et al. 2010; Xyrichis et al. 2018):

> Patients, clients and service users frequently have conditions that have multiple causes and require multiple treatments from a range of health and social care professions with different skills and expertise. As it is unusual for one profession to deliver a complete episode of care in isolation, good quality care depends upon professions working together in interprofessional teams. (Reeves et al. 2010, p. 13)

Teamwork in IPC teams is described as "a type of work which involves different health and/or social professions who share a team identity and work closely together in an integrated and interdependent manner to solve problems and deliver services" (Reeves et al. 2010, p 8). IPC team members may include physicians, nurses, medical assistants, social workers, psychologists, pharmacists, physical and rehabilitative therapists (physical, occupational, speech roles), dieticians, and other allied health professionals (Gergerich et al. 2018; Rice et al. 2010; Seaton et al. 2020). IPC teams may also include podiatrists, dieticians, orthoptists, radiologists, medical scientists, and exercise physiologists (Slade et al. 2018). In addition to teams, primary healthcare centers have been established to provide the opportunity to prevent, delay, and reduce the progression of chronic disease through shared responsibility, accountability, coordination, communication, cooperation, assertiveness, autonomy, mutual trust, and respect among practitioners (Seaton et al. 2020; Lizarondo et al. 2016; McInnes et al. 2015; Ontario College of Family Physicians 2000). However, the effectiveness of the integration and collaboration in PHCs depends on whether the professionals who are physically colocated continue to work as separate providers or strive to understand each other's professional roles and address power imbalances (Bonciani et al. 2018; Gergerich et al. 2018; Xyrichis et al. 2018; Tang et al. 2013). Research into the elements required for effective IPC has identified the importance of a range of elements that include identification of a shared purpose, philosophy and processes, the establishment of clear communication, and agreement on issues related to governance, power, autonomy, decision-making, and financial considerations (Xyrichis et al. 2018; Seaton et al. 2020).

In summary, while IPC has been promoted, there is little evidence that efforts to achieve IPC have resulted in effective, sustainable integration of the professions. Instead, demarcations and hierarchies between professions remain a dominant feature, entrenched by top-down decision-making processes that discourage shared values and decision-making, and differential funding between professions (Cunningham et al. 2012; Reeves et al. 2017; Evans et al. 2013, p. 127). Given this, the need to focus on educating a new generation of collaboration-ready practitioners through interprofessional education opportunities has been the subject of much discussion.

4.3 Interprofessional Education (IPE)

The World Health Organization (WHO 2010, p. 7) defined interprofessional education (IPE) as "when students from two or more professions learn about, from and with each other in order to enable effective collaboration and improve health outcomes." Both Thistlethwaite (2015) and Schaik et al. (2015) explained that the aim of IPE is to ensure the graduation of collaboration-ready practitioners.

Curriculum design for healthcare has traditionally focused on the development of technical expertise required by specific professions (Thistlethwaite 2015). Attempts to increase collaboration between the professions by changing the educational focus have led to the extension of curriculum beyond technical competency to include interprofessional competency and skills (Schaik et al. 2015). Curriculum designed for IPE aims to extend graduates' thinking and social skills to enable them to "identify and define problems and to establish and manage in an evolving context" (Hartviksen et al. 2018, p. 2). This discourse led to the development of a global Framework for Action on Interprofessional Education and Collaborative Practice by the World Health Organization (WHO 2010).[1] The preface of this framework identifies the need to:

(i) Prepare a 'collaborative practice-ready' health workforce to respond to local health needs.
(ii) Ensure that students graduate with an understanding of the range of skills needed for collaboration for working in teams that includes understanding each other's roles and responsibilities, communicating effectively, and critically reflecting for learning, building relationships, and engaging in ethical practice that acknowledges each other's views.
(iii) Support collaborative practice through a focus on bringing together multiple health workers from different professional backgrounds to work with patients, families, carers, and communities to deliver the highest quality of care.
(iv) Provide a mechanism for health policymakers to encourage and shape IPE and collaborative practice.

The preface highlights the importance of establishing the following:

(i) Supportive management practices and champions of collaboration.
(ii) Resolution to change the culture and attitudes of health workers.
(iii) Willingness to update, renew, and revise existing curricula.
(iv) Legislation to eliminate barriers to collaborative practice.

The framework recommends that key stakeholders design customized implementation approaches through the:

(i) Agreement on a common vision and purpose for interprofessional education.
(ii) Development of curricula in accord with principles of good educational practice.
(iii) Provision of organizational support, including adequate financial resources and time.
(iv) Inclusion of IPE in health worker training programs.
(v) Ensurance of staff competence and expertise in developing, delivering, and evaluating IPE.

[1] Given the global importance of the IPE framework, its main elements are summarized with some detail.

The framework identifies actions to advance collaborative practices that include:

(i) Structures and processes that promote shared decision-making.
(ii) Regular communication and community involvement.
(iii) A built environment that promotes, fosters, and extends interprofessional collaborative practice both within and across service agencies.
(iv) Personnel policies that recognize and support collaborative practice.
(v) Fair and equitable remuneration models.
(vi) A delivery model that allows adequate time and space for staff to focus on interprofessional collaboration and delivery of care.
(vii) Governance models that establish teamwork and shared responsibility for healthcare service delivery between team members as the normative practice.

Finally, the framework recommends that actions for collaboration be supported by the following:

(i) Systems to build workforce capacity at national and local levels.
(ii) Accreditation standards for health worker education programs that include clear evidence of IPE.
(iii) Policy and regulatory frameworks that support educators and health workers to promote and practice collaboratively, including new and emerging roles and models of care.
(iv) Frameworks and allocation of funding for clear interprofessional outcomes as part of lifelong learning for the health workforce.
(v) An environment in which to share best practices from workforce planning, financing, funding, and remuneration that support IPE and collaborative practice.

While the IPE Framework provides this detailed list of how to structure IPE, it is left to practitioners to design programs. Bridges et al. (2011) designed three models based on the IPE Framework to educate students in collaboration:

(i) Curriculum designed for cross-discipline courses of study.
(ii) Experiential learning opportunities or simulations designed to engage students in collaborative team interactions.
(iii) Communication, service learning, and assessment inclusive of evidence-based practice and quality improvement.

Bridges et al. went on to claim that these models would engage students in developing skills in responsibility, accountability, coordination, communication, cooperation, assertiveness, autonomy, and mutual trust and respect. They stated that the models have been assessed as developing students who are more likely to become "collaborative interprofessional team members who show respect and positive attitudes towards each other and work towards improving patient outcomes" (Bridges et al. 2011, pp. 1–2). However, these claims have been questioned by research into students' engagement in experiential (problem-based) learning in practice settings such as hospitals, primary practice, and community health. O'Leary et al. (2019) found that while students involved in practice-based teams of two or more professions did develop collaboration skills, this was not sustained past the learning experience (O'Leary et al. 2019). Factors that have been identified as limiting long-term collaboration include the following:

(i) The inability of learning environments to fully replicate the complexities of practice environments (Mink et al. 2021).
(ii) The continued existence of hierarchies between professions (Abu-Rish et al. 2012).
(iii) The lack of educational training of clinicians supervising student practice, particularly when tackling sensitive issues such as professional stereotypes and role boundaries.
(iv) The influence of the separate competencies required by specific regulatory bodies (O'Leary et al. 2020).

4.4 Discussion

In summary, despite attempts to encourage greater integration and collaboration between the healthcare professions through IPE, once practitioners are in professional practice, collaboration tends to become limited by the predominant hierarchical culture (Abu-Rish et al. 2012). Gergerich et al. (2018, p. 528) concluded that "even when education involves multiple professions and takes place face-to-face, if issues of hierarchy go unresolved, it could impact the effectiveness of interprofessional collaboration." Similarly, Grace (2021, p. 780) concluded that more profound change to practices and processes is needed to embrace an approach that encourages "networks of skilled individuals, rather than a set of skills possessed by a single individual." This requires IPE that consists of "modules that provide new skills and knowledge…as new career paths in healthcare emerge." They proposed further change to include the establishment of the following:

(i) A community of educator networks at clinical sites to focus on "how people engage with rule-governing systems, and to use tools to achieve objectives in real-life circumstances" (O'Leary et al. 2020, p. 2).
(ii) Robust partnerships between universities and clinical educators in placements (O'Leary et al. 2021).

It is noteworthy that Buckland (2020) reported a different experience of medical students in the UK who worked closely (as volunteers) during the COVID-19 pandemic in local hospitals with health professionals. During this time, they shared activity and decisions. Students claimed that they had gained valuable experience in collaboration, because "by working closely with nurses, medical students gained practical understanding of the different roles within the hospital environment and [had] been involved in providing hand-on-care to patients" (Buckland 2020, p. 679). This experience suggests that further research using a similar model is needed.

Given the need for further research, the authors undertook a reflection on the implications of the proposals for change discussed above by mapping these against the 3P agencies of health and healthcare: Principles and Purposes (P1); People in Place (P2); and Practices and Processes (P3). The findings, identified in Table 4.1, suggest the need for future research to detail the changes needed, particularly in regard to the need for the following:

Table 4.1 The 3P Agencies of Health and Healthcare: mapping the implications of proposals for change in IPC and IPE

3P agencies of health and healthcare	IPC	IPE
P1 **Principles and Purposes**	Share philosophy, commitment, and values to identify clear goals	• Graduate collaborative practice-ready practitioners • Agree on a common vision • Adopt good educational practice
P2 **People and Place**	Engage physicians, nurses, medical assistants, and allied health professionals (social workers, psychologists, pharmacists, physical and rehabilitation therapists, dieticians) who • Develop mutual trust and respect • Agree on degree of autonomy and guidance, regulation, task independence, and/or interdependence • Encourage physical proximity (co-location)	Stakeholders, IP champions, and community representatives • Learn from each other • Change culture and attitudes of health workers
P3 **Practices and Processes (i)**	• Collaborate—Identify clear team roles • Share responsibility, accountability, and coordination • Develop interdependencies • Develop an agreed process and system for communication	• Establish structures and processes supportive of shared decision-making and teamwork • Design a supportive built environment • Design supportive personnel policies
P3 **Practices and Processes (ii)**	• Encourage frequent interactions • Coordinate work practices • Establish networks • Share finances equitably • Graduate students with PP competencies	• Build workforce capacity at national and local level • Ensure organizational support, including financial resources and time • Ensure educators' competence • Communicate regularly • Ensure fair and equitable remuneration • Focus on new skills for collaboration
P3 **Practices and Processes (iii)**	Use diagnostic tools	Create new accreditation standards that include evidence of IPE and lifelong learning

1. A shared philosophy, vision, values, and goals across healthcare professions and the means to graduate students as collaborative, practice-ready practitioners.
2. A focus on building trusting and respectful relationships between practitioners based on a commitment to shared context and culture, and the means to encourage commitment to learning from each other.
3. The design of practices and processes to support and encourage collaboration, to include commitment to, funding for, and assessment of collaboration, in teams.

4.5 Conclusion

In summary, while it has been acknowledged that collaboration for holistic health and healthcare requires greater integrated and collaboration between healthcare professions, there is little evidence of a move away from the traditional separation between the professions and sub professions. Attempts to develop IPC and IPE to graduate new healthcare professionals as collaboration-ready practitioners have had little sustained success. Identification of the implications for the three agencies of health and healthcare revealed the need for further research. The implications of these findings are considered further in later chapters.

4.6 Reflective Pause Point

1. From your experience of healthcare, either as a professional or as a patient, can you recall an example of an integrated approach in which more than one health professional collaborated?
2. From your experience as a healthcare educator or student, what challenges do graduates face to be ready for work as collaborative cross-discipline practitioners?

References

Abu-Rish E, Kim S, Choe L et al (2012) Current trends in interprofessional education of health sciences students: a literature review. J Interprof Care 26(6):444–451. https://doi.org/10.3109/13561820.2012.715604

Beirne M (2017) The reforming appeal of distributed leadership. British Journal of Healthcare Management, 23(6): 262–270

Bonciani N, Schäfer W, Barsanti S et al (2018) The benefits of co-location in primary care practices: the perspectives of general practitioners and patients in 34 countries. BMC Health Serv Res 18(132):3–22. https://doi.org/10.1186/s12913-018-2913-4

Bridges DR, Davidson RA, Odegard PS et al (2011) Interprofessional collaboration: three best practice models of interprofessional education. Med Educ Online 16. https://doi.org/10.3402/meo.v16i0.6035. PMID: 21519399
Buckland R (2020) Medical student volunteering during COVID-19: lessons for future interprofessional practice. J Interprof Care 34(5):679–681. https://doi.org/10.1080/13561820.2020.1822790
Burns LR, Goldsmith JC, Sen A (2013) Horizontal and vertical integration of physicians: a tale of two tails. Adv Health Care Manag 15(39):117–161. https://doi.org/10.1108/s1474-8231(2013)0000015007. PMID: 24749211
Cunningham FC, Ranmuthugala G, Plumb J et al (2012) Health professional networks as a vector for improving healthcare quality and safety; a systematic review. BMJ Qual Saf 21:239–249
D'Amour D, Ferrada-Videla M, San Martin RL et al (2005) The conceptual basis for interprofessional collaboration: core concepts and theoretical frameworks. J Interprof Care 19(suppl 1):116–131
Evans J, Baker G, Berta W et al (2013) The evolution of integrated health strategies. Adv Health Care Manag 15:125–161. https://doi.org/10.1108/s1474-8231(2013)0000015007. PMID: 24749211
Fox A, Reeves S (2015) Interprofessional collaborative patient centred care: a critical exploration of two related discourses. J Interprof Care 29(2):113–118. https://doi.org/10.3109/13561820.2014.954284
Gergerich E, Boland D, Scott MA (2018) Hierarchies in interprofessional training. J Interprof Care 33(5):528–535. https://doi.org/10.1080/13561820.2018.1538110
Grace S (2021) Models of interprofessional education for healthcare students: a scoping review. J Interprof Care 35(5):771–783. https://doi.org/10.1080/13561820.2020.1767045
Hall P (2005) Interprofessional teamwork: professional cultures as barriers. J Interprof Care 19(sup1):188–196. https://doi.org/10.1080/13561820500081745
Hartviksen T, Sjolie B, Aspfors J et al (2018) Healthcare middle managers' experiences developing leadership capacity and capability in a public funded learning network. BMC Health Sci Res 18:433. https://doi.org/10.1186/s12913-018-3259-7
Illich I (1981) Limits to medicine: medical nemesis. Penguin, London
Kates N, Craven M (1999) Family medicine and psychiatry. Opportunities for sharing mental health care. Can Fam Physician 45(2561–3):72–74
Kinnaman M, Bleich M (2004) Collaboration: aligning resources to create and sustain partnerships. J Prof Nurs 20:310–322
Lancaster G, Kolakowsky-Hayner S, Kovacich J et al (2015) Interdisciplinary communication and collaboration among physicians, nurses, and unlicensed assistive personnel. J Nurs Scholarsh 47(3):275–284. https://doi.org/10.1111/jnu.12130
Lizarondo L, Turnbull C, Kroon T et al (2016) Allied health: integral to transforming health. Aust Health Rev 40(2):194–204. https://doi.org/10.1071/AH15044
McInnes S, Peters K, Bonney A et al (2015) An integrative review of facilitators and barriers influencing collaboration and teamwork between general practitioners and nurses working in general practice. J Adv Nurs 71(9):1973–1985. https://doi.org/10.1111/jan.2015.71.issue-9
McKimm J (2011) Leading for collaboration and partnership working. In: Swanwick T, McKimm J (eds) ABC of clinical leadership. Wiley Blackwell, Chichester, pp 44–49
Mink J, Mitzkat A, Krug K et al (2021) Impact of an interprofessional training ward on interprofessional competencies—a quantitative longitudinal study. J Interprof Care 35(5):751–759. https://doi.org/10.1080/13561820.2020.1802240
O'Leary N, Salmon N, Clifford A et al (2019) Bumping along: a qualitative metasynthesis of challenges to interprofessional placements. Med Educ 53(9):903–915
O'Leary N, Salmon N, Clifford A (2020) It benefits patient care: the value of practice-based IPE in healthcare curriculum. BMC Med Educ 20:42. https://doi.org/10.1186/s12909-020-02356-
O'Leary N, Salmon N, Clifford AM (2021) Inside-out: normalising practice-based IPE. Adv in Health Sci Educ 26:653–666. https://doi.org/10.1007/s10459-020-10017-8

Ontario College of Family Physicians (2000) Implementation strategies: Collaboration in primary care—family doctors and nurse practitioners delivering shared care. https://ocfp.on.ca/docs/public-policy-documents/implementation-strategies-collaboration-in-primary-care—family-doctors-nurse-practitioners-deliveringshared-care.pdf

Ponte PR, Conlin G, Conway JB et al (2003) Making patient-centred care come alive. J Nurs Admin 33: 82–90

Reddy S (2017) Exploration of funding models to support hybridisation of Australian primary health care organisations. J Prim Health Care 9(3):208–211. https://doi.org/10.1071/HC17014

Reeves S, Lewin S, Espin S et al (2010) Interprofessional teamwork for health and social care. Wiley-Blackwell, Sussex

Reeves S, Pelone F, Harrison R et al (2017) Interprofessional collaboration to improve professional practice and healthcare outcomes. Cochrane Database Syst Rev 6:CD000072. https://doi.org/10.1002/14651858.CD000072.pub3

Rice K, Zwarenstein M, Conn LG et al (2010) An intervention to improve interprofessional collaboration and communications: a comparative qualitative study. J Interprof Care 24(4):350–361. https://doi.org/10.3109/13561820903550713

Schaik S, Plant J, O'Brien B (2015) Challenges of interprofessional team training: a qualitative analysis of residents' perceptions. Edu Health 28(1):52–57. https://doi.org/10.4103/1357-6283.161883

Schroeder RE, Morrison EE, Cavanaugh C et al (1999) Improving communication among health professionals through education: a pilot study. J Health Admin Edu 17:175–198

Seaton J, Jones A, Johnston C et al (2020) Allied health professionals' perceptions of interprofessional collaboration in primary health care: an integrative review. J Interprof Care 35(2):217–228. https://doi.org/10.1080/13561820.2020.1732311

Silver J, Baima J (2013) Cancer prehabilitation: an opportunity to decrease treatment-related morbidity, increase cancer treatment options, and improve physical and psychological health outcomes. Am J Phys Med Rehabil 92(8):715–727. https://doi.org/10.1097/PHM.0b013e31829b4afe

Slade S, Philip K, Morris M (2018) Frameworks for embedding a research culture in allied health practice: a rapid review. Health Research Policy and Systems 16:29. https://doi.org/10.1186/s129061-018-0304

Steele S, Toribio J-A, Mor SM (2022) A vision of a One Health system for Australia: on the need to rethink our health system. Medical Journal of Australia. John Wiley & Sons Australia, Ltd on behalf of AMPCo Pty Ltd.

Tang CJ, Chan SW, Zhou WT et al (2013) Collaboration between hospital physicians and nurses: an integrated literature review. Int Nurs Rev 60(3):291–302. https://doi.org/10.1111/inr.12034

Tasselli S (2015) Social networks and interprofessional knowledge transfer: the case of healthcare professionals. Organ Stud 36(7):841–872

Thistlethwaite JE (2015) Interprofessional education: implications and development for medical education. Educación Médical 6(1):68–73. https://doi.org/10.1016/j.edumed.2015.04.007

Way D, Jones L, Busing N (2000) Implementation strategies, collaboration in primary care—family doctors & nurse practitioners delivering shared care. Ontario College of Family Physicians, Toronto

WHO, United Nations Children's Fund (UNICEF) (2020) Operational framework for primary health care. Technical Series on Primary Health Care

Witz A (1992) Professions and patriarchy. Routledge, London

World Health Organization (WHO) (2010) Framework for action on interprofessional education and collaborative practice. https://www.who.int/publications/i/item/framework-for-action-on-interprofessional-education-collaborative-practice

Xyrichis A, Reeves S, Zwarenstein M (2018) Examining the nature of interprofessional practice: an initial framework validation and creation of the InterProfessional Activity Classification Tool (InterPACT). J Interprof Care 32(4):416–425. https://doi.org/10.1080/13561820.2017.1408576

Chapter 5
Integrating Patients

Sandra Jones and Dein Vindigni OAM

Abstract The aim of this chapter is to identify proposals for changes for health professionals and patients to co-design and co-create health and healthcare. The chapter presents discourse on several proposals for change, including: integrative healthcare, adaptive health practice, patient-centered care (patient voice and patients as partners), and relationship-centered care. The discussion is complemented by the authors reflections upon these proposals aimed to identify the implications of each for each of the 3P agencies of health and healthcare: Principles and Purposes (P1); People in Place (P2); and Practices and Processes (P3).

5.1 Introduction

As the complex needs of patients have increased, so has the breadth and depth of knowledge required by both healthcare practitioners and patients. Bridges et al. (2011, p. 1) stated that "today's patients have complex health needs and typically require more than one discipline to address issues regarding their health status." In urging the adoption of primary healthcare (PHC), the World Health Organization (WHO) opted for the adoption of "a whole-of-society approach designed to effectively organize and strengthen national health systems to bring services for health and wellbeing closer to communities" (WHO, https://www.who.int/health-topics/primary-health-care#tab=tab_1). PHC outlines a vision for healthcare built on three components: i) providing integrated health services to meet people's health needs throughout their lives; ii) addressing the broader determinants of health through multisectoral policy and action; and iii) empowering individuals, families, and communities to take charge of their own health. This chapter focuses on the third of

S. Jones (✉)
Business and Law College, RMIT University, Melbourne, VIC, Australia

D. Vindigni OAM
STEM College, RMIT University, Melbourne, VIC, Australia
e-mail: dein.vindigni@rmit.edu.au

S. Jones, D. Vindigni OAM (eds.), *Health and Healthcare in Complexity*,
https://doi.org/10.1007/978-981-96-0515-6_5

these components, actively engaging patients, communities, and other stakeholders in the co-creation of a holistic approach (WHO and United Nations Children's Fund 2020). A holistic approach is in keeping with enabling people to increase control over, and improve their health (WHO 1998, https://www.who.int/health-topics/health-promotion#tab=tab_1). Actively engaging patients in their own health differs from traditional medical principles and practices that view patients simply as recipients of technical solutions rather than as active participants (Pomey et al. 2015; Thygeson 2013). Traditional thinking has led to the design of practices and processes that assume the superiority of technical (medical) solutions over patient expertise (Noyes 2021). In its place, there is need for a more inclusive and engaged approach. This chapter discusses four approaches designed to integrate patients: Integrative Healthcare; Adaptive Health Practice; Patient-Centered Care and Relationship-Centered Care.

5.2 Integrative Healthcare

Integrative healthcare (IHC), often referred to as integrative medicine, has been described as a more holistic approach to health and healthcare that places the patient at the center. Bell et al. (2002) defined IHC as a transformative, higher-order system of care that emphasizes the wellness and healing of the entire person (including biopsycho-socio-spiritual dimensions) as a primary goal. Coulter et al. (2010, p. 691) emphasized that IHC must be underpinned by shared practice, which they defined as "a new form of medical practice involving shared management of the patient, shared patient care, shared practice guidelines, and shared common values and goals (i.e., to treat the person in a 'whole-person' approach and not just the disease)."

Integrative healthcare can include biomedical, allied health, and complementary and alternative medicine (Hollenberg 2006); chiropractic, naturopathic, acupuncture, and massage therapists; holistic nurse practitioners; and, in some cases, spiritual healers and touch therapists (Coulter et al. 2010). Given the number of different disciplines involved, IHC requires collaboration. Boon et al. (2009, p. 3) defined collaboration as "an inter-professional process for communication and decision-making that enables the separate and shared knowledge and skills of health care providers to synergistically influence the client/patient care provided."

IHC has been extensively trialed in Canada, the USA, and China. In Canada, IHC is chiefly provided as a private service paid for by patients/clients, rather than as part of public health services. From their research into IHC practices in Canada, Boon et al. (2004) identified four elements that constitute a framework for IHC:

1. Philosophy and values. IHC is focused on healing rather than disease and thus engages the mind, spirit, and community as well as the body, through a partnership between patient and practitioner. IHC is thus seen as an innately interdisciplinary and nonhierarchical approach in which complementary medicine (previously also known as alternative medicine) engages with conventional med-

icine to provide a seamless continuum of decision-making and patient-centered care and support.
2. Structure, or sociopolitical context. IHC employs a collaborative team approach guided by consensus-building, mutual respect, and a shared vision of healthcare that permits each practitioner and patient to contribute their particular knowledge and skills within the context of a shared, synergistically charged plan of care.
3. Process, or professional practice. IHC focuses on communicating and decision-making that enables care providers' to share knowledge and skills to synergistically influence client/patient care. It seeks, through a partnership of patient and practitioners, to treat the whole person, to assist the innate healing properties of each person, and to promote health and wellness as well as the prevention of disease.
4. Outcomes. IHC is focuses on expanding measures of output to include measures of the collective effect of the individual practice.

Despite the holistic, integrative intent of IHC, experience of the degree of integration has varied. In their early research, Boon et al. (2004) found that integration was greater at the consumer (patient) level but that it decreased incrementally across the practitioner, clinic, and institutional levels, to be nonexistent at the professional/regulatory body level and in health policy. In their later research, Boon et al. (2009, p. 719) found that:

> any perceived loss of autonomy by any participants was generally considered to be less desirable…participants generally described a model of professions working closely together in the delivery of care (i.e. collaboration) but not being subsumed into a single organizational framework (i.e. integration).

Accordingly, they argued that IHC requires the following:

1. A mix of components that include the ability for participants to work, together with different disciplines, interdependently, cooperatively, including sharing information, and with mutual respect.
2. A decision-making process to enable agreement on five conflicting variables: (i) common governance or maintenance of professional autonomy; (ii) common organization and structures or independent administrative functions and structures; (iii) blurred or separate roles, responsibilities, identity, and professional boundaries; (iv) shared or common patients and shared or mutual roles; and (v) whether collaboration or integration is the aim.

To these elements, Gaboury et al. (2009) added that collaboration in IHC needs to be supported by:

(i) Dual education and training aimed at raising the awareness of new entrants and existing practitioners to reduce barriers and conflicts between healthcare paradigms.
(ii) Social, professional, and financial processes that support the evolution of relationships between IHC team members.
(iii) Intellectual stimulation and personal growth to keep practitioners interested in working in an IHC clinic.

5.3 Adaptive Health Practice

Adaptive health practice (AHP) grew from consideration of the need for healthcare to develop as an adaptive state, unique to each person (Sturmberg et al. 2010; Thygeson et al. 2010). It is based in the principle that healthcare systems need to change from "illness centred to health-centred; provider-centred to patient-centred; and reductionist, technical medicine to holistic, adaptive medicine" (Thygeson 2013, p. 661). AHP applies the concepts of adaptive leadership theory to clinical-patient partnerships, in which leadership is regarded as an activity to explain how organizations and human beings interact as part of a complex adaptive system (Heifetz 1994). The aim is to "address the environmental, social and behavioural determinants of their (and our) health" (Thygeson 2013, p. 662). The goals of AHP (Thygeson 2013, p. 661) include the following:

> to help patients be healthy, resilient and maximally autonomous producers of their own health; to increase productivity and reduce community sick-care costs due to reduced morbidity and more efficient return to health; and to provide a sustainable, satisfying professional life for providers.

Adaptation to challenges that typically arise are explained as "when substantial change in a person's internal state or environment causes performance deterioration or creates a gap between the way things are and the way they need to be" (Thygeson et al. 2010, p. 1010). Responding to these challenges requires active participation by patients that goes beyond technical solutions where "both the problem and the potential solution can be easily identified...[and] amenable to expertise" (Thygeson et al. 2010, p. 1010). This requires active patient participation to empower patient 'voice' that supplements surgical and other therapeutic procedures and the prescription of medications. This acknowledges that, on the one hand, patients recognize the need for change and a willingness to learn new behaviors, beliefs, and attitudes and abandon old ones that no longer serve them. Thygeson et al. (2010, p. 1010) described this as "to survive and thrive in the face of an adaptive challenge, people must adapt" (p. 1010). On the other hand, it requires health professionals to provide leadership to combine clinicians' technical expertise with patients' experience-based expertise to "make explicit our need to actively address providers' and patients' interdependence" (Thygeson et al. 2010, p. 1012).

For AHP to be effective, there is need to move away from assumptions that underpin three key mental models of modern medical practice (Thygeson 2013, pp. 669–670):

(i) That healing is something that physicians 'do to' patients rather than that patients do to themselves.
(ii) That medical technology can promote health and cure disease.
(iii) That patient behavior is difficult, if not impossible, to affect.

These assumptions need to be replaced by new insights:

(i) That health systems can be viewed as emergent phenomena that result from repetitive iteration of 'simple rules' built into the system structure.
(ii) That intervention must occur at multiple levels of the system to effect lasting beneficial change by balancing feedback loops.
(iii) That the shared goal of a therapeutic process and nonhierarchical relationships based on trust and mutual regard must be adopted.

The change required to implement adaptive health practice includes an increase in both education and communication. Learning is needed in the science of behavior change, the role of social networks, and the influence of social and environmental factors on health "at the very least to leverage the most basic and potentially the most important, social network intervention…the therapeutic clinician-patient relationship" (Thygeson 2013, p. 669). This includes change to:

(i) Adopt principles and philosophy of care so that patients can make an informed decision about whether the healthcare practice's philosophy of care matches their own.
(ii) Design a plan of action based on a combination of physical examination of the patient and information on the patient's lifestyle, health and psychological outlook, social support, social networks, and environment.
(iii) Provide a clear distinction and explanation of the difference between technical (clinical) challenges and adaptive (patient) behavioral changes.
(iv) Design evaluation methods that are inclusive of assessment of the quality of the clinic-patient relationship.
(v) Develop a patient plan that is iterative and includes observation, interpretation, and intervention.

These changes presage a more patient-centered care approach.

5.4 Patient-Centered Care

Patient-centered care (PCC) first emerged as a concept in the late 1950s (Balint 1955). It was promoted as part of a holistic approach that views patients as biopsychosocial entities (Henbest and Stewart 1989), with lived experience that can complement medical expertise (Noyes 2021; Bridges et al. 2011). Its potential importance has grown as multiple components (agents) that contribute to health and healthcare have been recognized (Sturmberg et al. 2010). Sturmberg (2022, p. 2) summarized this as the need for "constant weaving together of the often seemingly unconnected pieces of history with clinical findings, and the management of uncertainties, patient understandings, anxieties and treatment choices."

Implementing PCC requires change at all levels of healthcare (Sturmberg et al. 2010). At the macro level, there is need for national support for policy that identifies an improved health experience as the system's central goal and has strong integrated primary care as the key strategy by which to achieve it. At the meso level, it requires ensuring that practices and services are equitably distributed in the community to allow easy access to healthcare for all. At the microlevel, it requires practice and service-based teams to assess patient health needs. Underpinning this is the need to understand the connections and system dynamics between these levels (Sturmberg 2022), together with the active involvement of patients in "developing, prioritizing and implementing patient-reported and other quality indicators for use at the aggregated service user level in quality improvement, public reporting, research, accreditation, certification and payment within health systems" (de Bienassis et al. 2021, p. 114).

Discourse upon implementing PCC has had two main foci: patient voice and patients-as-partners.

5.4.1 *Patient Voice*

Patients, it is argued, are "in a unique position to contribute to the quality of healthcare since they are the ones who experience the whole episode of care from primary care in communities through hospital care to rehabilitation and follow up in general practice" (Mainz et al. 2022, p. 111). Speaking as a physician, Hannan (2022, p. i) observed that "it was when they told their unique life journeys in the presence of another person who was 'listening' and not just hearing the words, the healing processes began." As a 'listening' physician, Hannan describes himself as "not the 'saviour', but the person who provided a *time space* in which they could be heard and believed" (p. 2).

Patient voice has been made possible through the development of systems such as patient-reported experience measures (PREMs) and patient-reported outcomes measures (PROMs). Both systems enable the collection of feedback about symptoms, physical functioning, and/or health-related quality of life. This offers the potential to capture "how a patient feels and functions during routine care, providing information that is useful to the patient themselves with regard to treatment choices, to the health-care professional and to the health service provider" (Calvert et al. 2019, p. 732). However, while it is claimed that these systems have had a positive impact, Dean et al. (2017, p. 700) counter claimed that simply enabling patients' voices to be heard has limited impact away from the "paternalistic health care professional to an empowered patient."

5.4.2 *Patients-as-Partners (PP)*

The limitation of patient voice has led to discourse on patients-as-partners (PP) designed to actively engage patients in contributing their experiential knowledge of their health. This can be achieved by patients becoming members of a team that involves them in a variety of activities varying from research into the disease affecting them and the impact of treatment, to patient identification of their priorities for treatment, patient-to-patient peer support, patient assessment of quality of care, patient setting of health policy agendas, and the development of coordinated care plans between professions (Dean et al. 2017; Pomey et al. 2015). In addition, healthcare organization need to embed the time taken to engage in PP into workflows and daily schedules (Busari et al. 2017; Lackie and Tomblin Murphy 2020; Pannick et al. 2014).

Not surprisingly, given the degree of change and commitment to change required, there are few examples of success. One significant example is the global co-creation process that developed measures of patients' experiences of mental healthcare delivery (World Health Organization, World Bank Group and OECD 2018). Vanstone et al. (2023, p. 2) stated:

> although there are many papers describing patient partnership, few move beyond single-site descriptions of involvement.... As a result...there has been little synthesis to describe the role of patient partners across multiple health system domains.... We have no consolidated understanding of how the patient partner role has been defined and how these individuals have been engaged, in what roles.

Responsibility for the limited success of these initiatives has been attributed to reticence by both professionals and patients. On the one hand, professionals prioritize their technical (medical) solutions over patient expertise. Soklaridis et al. (2017, p. 124) stated that "healthcare professionals can't feel comfortable admitting when they lack knowledge without losing the client's/patient's confidence." On the other hand, patients often lack health literacy (knowledge, skills, and confidence) and continue to rely on health professionals, rather than accepting responsibility for taking action to improve personal and community health by changing personal lifestyles and living conditions (Pomey et al. 2015; https://www.who.int/activities/improving-health-literacy).

This limited success of PP leads us to discuss the experience of relationship-centered care.

5.5 Relationship-Centered Care

Relationship-centered care (RCC) is a model of care that seeks to articulate both:

> the doctors' and patients' agendas to find and explore common ground and to explore both the disease and illness experience...not just on technically appropriate transactions within these relationships. (Beach et al. 2005, S3)

Beach et al. (2005, S4) claimed that RCC is intrinsic to healthcare as long as it adheres to four foundational principles to:

(i) View each patient as a unique individual with their own experiences, values, and perspectives.
(ii) Challenge the dominant notion of detached concern in healthcare by recognizing the effect of emotions.

(iii) Recognize that interrelationship for reciprocal influence occurs across and between time, space, and content.
(iv) Acknowledge that relationships are morally valuable within themselves (rather than simply being of financial benefit).

In practice, RCC requires an emphasis on three factors:

(i) Communication to be viewed as "an interactive process that is dependent on the efforts of both participants" (Beach et al. 2005, S6).
(ii) Participant contribution of knowledge, skills, attitudes, actions, and behaviors to acknowledge the importance of reciprocity, mutual respect, and actions cognizant of patients' individual values, expectations, preferences, and backgrounds and the fluid nature of relationships that change over time as circumstances change (Beach et al. 2005).
(iii) Shared decision-making (Barry and Edgman-Levitan 2012).

5.6 Discussion

Empowering individuals, families, and communities to actively contribute to managing their individual health requires a paradigm shift by both the patient and the health professionals. This is in contrast to approaches to Indigenous health in which the self is seen as linked to body, mind, and emotions; family, kinship, and community; culture and country and spirit, and spirituality and ancestors (Gee et al. 2014).[1] Given the need for further research, the authors undertook a reflection on the implications of proposals for change discussed above for the 3P agencies of health and healthcare: Principles and Purposes (P1); People in Place (P2); and Practices and Processes (P3). The findings, identified in Table 5.1, reveal the need for further research to detail the changes needed to achieve the following:

1. Common commitment to a person-centered health approach that encourages patients to engage in codesign and co-creation of actions for heath and healthcare.
2. Collaboration between health professionals and patients to share both clinical expertise and the lived patient experience.
3. Practices and processes to develop reciprocal relationships through improved communication for collaboration that complements physical examination.
4. Skills to increase health literacy of patients.

[1] This is explained further in Chap. 11.

Table 5.1 The 3P Agencies of Health and Healthcare: mapping the implications of proposals for change to promote patient integration

3P agencies of health and healthcare	IHC/AHP	PCC Patient voice, PP	RCC
P1 Principles and Purposes	Agreement on a common goal of healing and wellness of entire person rather than illness	Codesign and co-create healthcare	Uniqueness of each patient ('dimension of personhood')
P2 People in Place	• Shared principles and philosophy of care inclusive of the quality of clinical-patient relationship • Collaboration between health professionals and patients based on consensus and mutual respect	Patients (family and community) contribute experiential knowledge	Patients and practitioners share combination of the importance of 'detached concern' and emotions
P3 Practices and Processes (i)	• Patient-centered teams • Distinction between patients' adaptive (experiential) knowledge and professionals' technical (clinical) • Action-based plans to share information on patients' lifestyles as well as physical examination	Patients and professionals develop opportunities for reciprocal relationships through increases in health literacy	Develop opportunities for reciprocal relationships
P3 Practices and Processes (ii)	• Structures to support collaboration • Processes to support communication • Dual education	Communication to be reciprocal and not limited to 'voice'.	Communication, accompanied by shared decision-making, central the interactive process
P3 Practices and Processes (iii)	• Measures of output to include personal growth, intellectual stimulation, and the collective effect of individual practice • Inclusive, iterative approach to patient plan inclusive of observation, interpretation, and intervention	Build collaborative relationships that can be adjusted over time as circumstances change	Emergent-adjustment of the relationship over time as circumstances change

5.7 Conclusion

In summary, while it is acknowledged that a co-creational approach that involves patients and professionals is important to advance patient-professional partnerships in health and healthcare, evidence of successful change is limited. The implications for future healthcare practice are discussed in later chapters.

5.8 Reflective Pause Point

1. From your experience of health and healthcare, as either a professional or a patient, can you recall a situation in which the patient was engaged as co-designer and/or co-creator of their health and healthcare?
2. Reflecting on the contribution that patients can made, what knowledge and skills are required of patients to ensure the success of a PP relationship?

References

Balint M (1955) The doctor, his patient and the illness. Lancet 318:683

Barry MJ, Edgman-Levitan S (2012) Shared decision making—pinnacle of patient-centered care. N Engl J Med 366(9):780–781. https://doi.org/10.1056/NEJMp1109283. PMID: 2237596

Beach MC, Inui T, The Relationship-Centered Care Research Network (2005) Relationship-centered care. A constructive reframing, vol 21. J Gen Intern Med, pp S3–S8

Bell IR, Caspi O, Schwartz GER et al (2002) Integrative medicine and systemic outcomes research: issues in the emergence of new model for primary health care. Archives of Internal Medicine I 162:133–140

Boon H, Verhoef M, O'Hara (2004) Integrative healthcare: arriving at a working definition. Altern Ther Health Med 10(5):48–56

Boon H, Verhoef M, O'Hara D et al (2009) From parallel practice to integrative health care: a conceptual framework. BMC Health Serv Res 4:15

Bridges DR, Davidson RA, Odegard PS et al (2011) Interprofessional collaboration: three best practice models of interprofessional education. Med Educ Online 16. https://doi.org/10.3402/meo.v16i0.6035. PMID: 21519399; PMCID: PMC3081249

Busari JO, Moll FM, Duits AJ (2017) Understanding the impact of interprofessional collaboration on the quality of care: a case report from a small scale resource limited health care environment. J Multidiscip Healthc 10:227–234. https://doi.org/10.2147/jmdh.s14004

Calvert M, O'Connor D, Basch E (2019) Harnessing the patient voice in real-world evidence: the essential role of patient-reported outcomes. Nat Rev 18:731–732

Coulter I, Chorsan R, Crawford C et al (2010) Integrative health care under review: an emerging field. J Manip Physiol Ther 33(99):690–710

de Bienassis K, Kristensen S, Hewlett E et al (2021) Measuring patient voice matters: setting the scene for patient-reported indicators. Int J Qual Health Care 33:1–6

Dean S, Mathers J, Calvert M et al (2017) The patient is speaking: discovering the patient voice in ophthalmology. Br J Ophthalmol 101:700–708

Gaboury I, Bujold M, Bon H et al (2009) Interprofessional collaboration within Canadian integrative health clinics: key component. Soc Sci Med 69:707–715

Gee G, Dudgeon P, Schultz C, Hart A, Kelly K (2014) Social and emotional wellbeing and mental health: an aboriginal perspective. In: Dudgeon P, Milroy M, Walker R (eds) Working together: aboriginal and Torres Strait islander mental health and wellbeing principles and practice—revised edition, Chapter 4. Commonwealth of Australia, Canberra

Hannan T (2022) Heard, helped, healed. Hannan, Manufactured by Amazon.com.au. Sydney, NSW, Australia

Heifetz R (1994) Leadership without easy answers. Harvard University Press, Cambridge, MA

Henbest R, Stewart M (1989) Patient-centredness in the consultation: a method for measurement. Fam Pract 6:249–253

Hollenberg D (2006) Uncharted ground: patterns of professional interaction among complementary/alternative and biomedical practitioners in integrative health care settings. Soc Sci Med 62:731–744

Lackie K, Tomblin Murphy G (2020) The impact of interprofessional collaboration on productivity: important considerations in health human resources planning. Journal of Interprofessional Education & Practice 21:100375. https://doi.org/10.1016/j.xjep.2020.100375

Mainz J, Kristensen S, Roe D (2022) The power of the patient's voice in the modern healthcare system. Int J Quality Health Care 34:S1, ii1–S1, ii2. https://doi.org/10.1093/intqhc/mzac001

Noyes A (2021) Navigating the hierarchy: communicating power relationships in collaborative health care groups. Manag Commun Q 36(1):62–91

Pannick S, Beveridge I, Wachter RM et al (2014) Improving the quality and safety of care on the medical ward: a review and synthesis of the evidence base. Eur J Intern Med 25(10):874–887. https://doi.org/10.1016/j.ejim.2014.10.013

Pomey M-P, Ghadiri DP, Karazivan P, Fernandez N et al (2015) Patients as partners: a qualitative study of patients' engagement in their health care'. PLoS One 10(4):e0122499. https://doi.org/10.1371/journal.pone.0122499

Soklaridis S, Romano D, Fung WL-A et al (2017) Where is the client/patient voice in interprofessional healthcare team assessments? Findings from a one-day forum. J Interprof Care 31(1):122–124. https://doi.org/10.1080/13561820.2016.1233393

Sturmberg J (2022) There is more to 'making connections' to improve health outcomes. Glob Adv Health and Med 11:1–3

Sturmberg JP, O'Halloran DM, Martin CM (2010) People at the centre of complex adaptive health systems reform. MJA 193(8):474–478

Thygeson M (2013) Implementing adaptive health practice: a complexity-based philosophy of health care. In: Sturmberg JP, Martin CM (eds) Handbook of Systems and Complexity In Health. Springer Science + Business Media, New York, pp 661–684. https://doi.org/10.1007/978-1-4614-4998-0_38

Thygeson M, Morrissey L, Ulstad V (2010) Adaptive leadership and the practice of medicine: a complexity-based approach to reframing the doctor-patient relationship. J Eval Clin Pract 16(5):1009–1015

Vanstone M, Canfeld C, Evans C et al (2023) Towards conceptualizing patients as partners in health systems: a systematic review and descriptive synthesis. Health Res Policy Sys 21(12):1–14. https://doi.org/10.1186/s12961-022-00954-8

WHO (1998) Health topics, health promotion. https://www.who.int/health-topics/health-promotion#tab=tab_2. Accessed 09 Dec 2023

WHO & the United Nations Children's Fund (UNICEF) (2020) Operational Framework for Primary Health Care, Technical Series on Primary Health Care, WHO & the United Nations Children's Fund, ISBN (WHO) 978-92-4-001783-2 (electronic version)

World Health Organization, World Bank Group, OECD (2018) Delivering quality health services: a global imperative for universal health coverage. OECD Publishing, Geneva

Chapter 6
Access and Equity in Health and Healthcare

Salma Arabi and Ashleigh Moreland

Abstract The aim of this chapter is to identify the challenges of, and opportunities for, improving access and equity to healthcare in complexity. The chapter critically examines the multifaceted challenges of global healthcare access and equity, emphasizing the imperative of fair distribution. It navigates through factors such as socioeconomic status, systemic biases, and cultural influences, all contributing to persistent inequalities in healthcare accessibility worldwide, especially in developing countries. Strategies to enhance access and equity are explored, highlighting the health access framework's five crucial dimensions: availability, accessibility, accommodation, affordability, and acceptability. The authors advocate for a patient-centered perspective, acknowledging the hurdles posed by conflicting definitions in policy development. Diverse theories and frameworks, ranging from social justice to individual health behavior models, are introduced. This comprehensive approach identifies key dimensions influencing healthcare access. The chapter also delves into evolving healthcare landscapes in developing countries, discussing initiatives while recognizing the vital role played by informal healthcare providers in addressing access barriers. It emphasizes the necessity for cohesive, well-rounded strategies to overcome challenges in the global pursuit of equitable healthcare.

S. Arabi (✉)
STEM College, RMIT University, Melbourne, VIC, Australia

School of Nursing, Paramedicine, and Healthcare Sciences, Charles Sturt University, Wagga Wagga, Australia
e-mail: sarabi@csu.edu.au

A. Moreland
STEM College, RMIT University, Melbourne, VIC, Australia

S. Jones, D. Vindigni OAM (eds.), *Health and Healthcare in Complexity*,
https://doi.org/10.1007/978-981-96-0515-6_6

6.1 Introduction

A significant challenge affecting the provision of healthcare is ensuring equity of access for all people. The World Health Organization (WHO) describes equitable healthcare as the provision of health services and resources that are fairly distributed and accessible to all regardless of socioeconomic status, gender, ethnicity, or geographic location (WHO 2019). The United Nations (UN) states that access to healthcare is a fundamental human right (United Nations 1948). The WHO (1948) argues that unfavorable social conditions are known to have a deleterious influence on population health. However, access to healthcare remains unequal.

6.2 Causes of Unequal Access to, and Inequity in, Healthcare

In seeing the complex world as essentially interconnected, continually changing with the potential for new emergent futures, complexity science presents the opportunity to view access to, and equity in, health and healthcare from a different perspective. Boulton, Allen, and Bowman (2015, p. 3) claim that:

> [*the]* more naturalistic and organic idea of the 'world as complex' is closer to lived experience than the 'world as a machine'. If we understand its implications thoroughly, engaging with the complexities of the world or even just accepting that the world as complex may give better guidance as to how to gain success in our ventures and yet also engender a sustainable and equitable world.

For the individual, access to healthcare is influenced by a wide range of factors, including socioeconomic status, age, gender, race/ethnicity, geographic location, limited availability of healthcare services in the area, lack of health insurance, inability to pay for medical expenses, and lack of transportation (Berchick et al. 2019). Studies have shown that individuals from disadvantaged socioeconomic backgrounds are more likely to experience barriers to accessing healthcare than those from higher socioeconomic backgrounds (Marmot 2005). Older adults often require more healthcare services than younger individuals while also experiencing age-related health problems that require specialized care and are more likely to be uninsured or underinsured (Fronstin 2019). There are also systemic biases and discrimination against groups, such as racial and ethnic minorities, individuals with disabilities, and those who identify as LGBTQ+ (Artiga and Orgera 2020). In addition, there are cultural and social factors such as language barriers, lack of trust, and cultural beliefs or practices that may conflict with Western medical practices. These may affect an individual's willingness to seek and accept healthcare services.

Access to healthcare is influenced by its availability, accessibility, acceptability, and systemic barriers. Included in this are policies related to healthcare financing, delivery, and regulation, as well as broad social and economic policies that affect population health (Andermann 2016). Factors not directly related to health, such as access to transport, can also have an impact. People living in rural areas are often underserved by healthcare providers and may have to travel long distances to receive medical care. This can be especially challenging for those who do not have access to reliable transportation or who have limited financial resources (Hartley et al. 2020).

Access to, and inequity in, healthcare varies across countries (United Nations 2015). According to the WHO (2017), of the 1.6 billion people worldwide who lack access to basic healthcare services, over 80% live in developing countries (WHO 2017). This in turn leads to poor health outcomes and high morbidity and mortality. According to recent World Bank and WHO (2020) findings, life expectancy at birth in developed countries was 78 years compared to 64 years in developing countries.

Within developing countries, disparities in access to healthcare resources and services is a significant issue. The disparities are caused by a range of sociodemographic, economic, cultural, and political factors (Braveman and Gruskin 2003). These factors include poverty; lack of adequate healthcare infrastructure and resources, such as hospitals, clinics, medical supplies, and trained healthcare professionals; unequal distribution of wealth and resources; and issues related to gender and ethnicity (Orach 2009). In sub-Saharan Africa, for example, there is less than 1 doctor per 1000 people, compared to 1 doctor for every 250 people in developed countries (WHO 2023). In India, the wealthiest 10% of the population has access to more than 60% of the country's healthcare resources, while the poorest 40% has access to only 20% of the resources (OECD 2019). In many countries, women are more likely to face cultural norms and barriers and a lack of resources that prevent them from seeking medical care (Cousins 2020). In addition, women are likely to have less access to healthcare services, lower rates of health insurance coverage, and, as a result, higher morbidity and mortality rates than men (Manandhar et al. 2018). This experience is shared by many people from ethnic and minority groups, who are often marginalized and face discrimination.

Disparities in access and equity to healthcare also exist in developed countries. In the USA, for example, there is no government-provided free universal healthcare, with individuals having to purchase private health insurance or receive it as an employment benefit. The high cost of private health insurance and the significant proportion of the workforce whose jobs do not offer insurance benefits mean that many individuals cannot access it (Keisler-Starkey and Bunch 2022). In Australia, inequities of access for Indigenous people have resulted in an average life expectancy of Indigenous Aboriginal and Torres Strait Islander (ATSI) people that is 12.5 years less than that of the non-Indigenous population (National Indigenous Australian Agencies 2020).

Given the range of factors that cause inequality of access to healthcare, it is important to ensure that broad social and economic policies are culturally and linguistically appropriate so that patients are treated with respect and dignity (Curtis et al. 2019; Marmot 2020).

6.3 Strategies to Improve Access to, and Equity in, Healthcare

Developing strategies to improve access and equity to healthcare has been challenging given the many definitions and descriptions of access, accessibility, and equity regarding healthcare. On the one hand is the issue of accessibility to healthcare. Donabedian (1966) argued that accessibility is a "mediating factor" between the potential to produce services and the actual use of those services or the degree of adjustment based on population and healthcare resources (Donabedian 1966; Penchansky and Thomas 1981; Rapport et al. 2014; Shannon and Bashshur 1982). Bashshur et al. (1971) defined accessibility as a functional relationship between the population and medical facilities and resources that reflects the differential existence of obstacles, impediments, and difficulties or of factors that are facilitators for the beneficiaries of healthcare. Frenk (1992) posited that accessibility should be defined as the degree of adjustment between the characteristics of healthcare resources and those individuals who are in the process of seeking or obtaining care. He argues that the main limitations to accessibility are space and time, followed closely by environmental factors.

On the other hand is the issue of access to healthcare. Whitehead (1992) defined access as the physical ability to reach a healthcare provider, as measured by how easily individuals or communities can access clinicians, providers, or institutions. Culyer and Wagstaff (1993) defined access as the cost of receiving care that is imposed on an individual or community and whether they are able to meet that cost. Waters (2000) defined access as a combination of use of and need for care. Woldemichael et al. (2019) argued that access to healthcare encompasses the achievement of goals such as improved effectiveness and enhanced service quality. Advances in technology that have seen the introduction of telemedicine and telehealth, remote monitoring, electronic health records, and mobile health applications have expanded notions of access to healthcare to include the digital environment (American Medical Association 2020, HealthIT n.d.; WHO 2010).

Each of these different approaches have different impacts and solutions that result in an increased likelihood of confusion, inconsistent application, and inadequate understanding of underlying issues (Bright and Kuper 2018). The challenges for researchers, policymakers, and healthcare providers are that it becomes difficult to identify and address specific barriers and disparities in healthcare access (Donabedian 1966; Penchansky and Thomas 1981). This lack of clarity hinders policy development, resource allocation, and interventions aimed at improving access. In addition, incorrect definitions of access may lead to overlooking important dimensions of access to healthcare. For instance, if access is solely defined in terms of physical proximity to healthcare facilities, other critical factors such as financial affordability, cultural appropriateness, linguistic accessibility, or availability of specialized services may be neglected and result in incomplete interventions that fail to address the multifaceted nature of access barriers (Shannon and Bashshur 1982). Furthermore, inadequate definitions of access may perpetuate or exacerbate existing healthcare disparities and inequities. Failing to recognize and address disparities between different populations may hinder efforts to promote equity and to improve healthcare access for marginalized or vulnerable populations. This is because different population groups may face unique barriers to access based on their socioeconomic status, race, ethnicity, gender, or geographical location (Penchansky and Thomas 1981). The implications of incorrectly defining access to healthcare for policy are also significant, as they may be misguided or ineffective if they are based on incorrect definitions (Garzón-Orjuela et al. 2020). This lack of a single definition has resulted in the emergence of many theories and frameworks to explain and address access and equity in healthcare.

6.4 Theories and Frameworks of Access and Equity in Healthcare

Multiple theories and frameworks have been developed to address the issue of equity and access to healthcare, with the main difference being whether healthcare is viewed from either a social or an individual perspective. From a social perspective, the health equity and social justice framework (HESJF) identifies health disparities as the result of a complex interplay of social, economic, and political factors (Braveman and Gruskin 2003). The HESJF has been used to develop policies and programs aimed at reducing health disparities, including policies aimed at improving access to healthcare for underserved populations. The community health worker model proposes that community health workers can play a critical role in addressing health disparities by providing culturally appropriate healthcare services to underserved populations (Naimoli et al. 2014). The social determinants of health framework (SDHF) recognizes that health is influenced by a wide range of social factors, including poverty, education, employment, housing, and access to healthcare. The SDHF is grounded in the concept that addressing social factors is critical to improving health outcomes and reducing health inequities (Marmot 2020). The health belief model (HBM) focuses on why individuals may or may not engage in health behaviors (Rosenstock et al. 1988). This model has been used in a variety of settings to develop interventions aimed at increasing healthcare use among underserved populations. The HBM proposes that individuals are more likely to engage in health behaviors if they perceive themselves to be at risk of a health problem, recognize the benefits of positive health behavior as outweighing the costs, and believe they are capable of taking the required action. Finally, the capability approach proposes that healthcare should be designed to enable individuals to achieve their full potential, rather than simply providing them with basic healthcare services (Sen 1999).

A comprehensive framework that combines various views with the perspectives of both health professionals and patients is the health access framework (HAF) (Levesque et al. 2013). The HAF identifies five dimensions that affect access to healthcare:

1. Availability, which refers to the presence of necessary healthcare services and resources such as healthcare professionals, medical supplies, and technologies.
2. Accessibility, which refers to the physical and geographical aspects of accessing healthcare, such as proximity and transportation.
3. Accommodation, which refers to the fit between healthcare services and individual needs, including cultural and linguistic preferences.
4. Affordability, which refers to the financial costs of healthcare services and the ability of individuals to pay for them.
5. Acceptability, which refers to the extent to which healthcare services meet the expectations, beliefs, and values of individuals and communities.

These five dimensions correspond with abilities of individuals and/or communities that are based on five socioeconomic determinants: to perceive, to seek, to reach, to pay for, and to engage in healthcare. The HAF places emphasis on the need to expand beyond a simple supply-and-demand approach to understand the complexities of the journey involved in accessing healthcare services from a patient-centered perspective. The HAF encourages health researchers to look beyond the failure of healthcare systems as the sole barrier to access and presents the opportunity to examine broader barriers to access. Several studies have tested the validity and reliability of the HAF (Russell et al. 2019; Javanparast et al. 2018; Rodrigues et al. 2023). One study in Canada used the framework to evaluate access to mental health services, finding that the framework provides a comprehensive and useful approach to evaluate access (Russell et al. 2019). A study in Australia used the framework to evaluate access to primary care services, finding that the framework can identify areas of need and inform policy development (Javanparast et al. 2018). The HAF has also been used to evaluate the impact of interventions aimed at improving healthcare access. A study in Brazil used the HAF to evaluate a community-based intervention to improve access to prenatal care for low-income women (Rodrigues et al. 2023). The study found that the intervention improved several dimensions of healthcare access, including availability, accessibility, and acceptability. However, while the HAF provides a comprehensive understanding of access to healthcare, it focuses on individual factors and does not capture the broader social and structural determinants of access to healthcare.

6.5 Access and Equity Changes in Developing Countries

Proposals to address the challenges of access and equity in developing countries have included pressure on governments, nongovernmental organizations, and international organizations to promote more equitable healthcare. This has included pressure to invest in healthcare infrastructure and resources, to train and retrain healthcare professionals, to increase access to healthcare services, and to address the root causes of poverty, discrimination, and gender-based violence. Initiatives such as the Global Fund to Fight AIDS, Tuberculosis, and Malaria are an example of significant progress in providing access to healthcare services and to reduce health inequities in developing countries (The Global Fund 2022).

However, equitable healthcare provision remains a critical challenge, especially in developing countries, because of a continuing lack of resources and geographical dispersion. In addition, while developing countries account for 51% of the population, they only contribute 4.2% to global spending on health (WHO 2022). One of the means used in developing countries to address barriers to access healthcare is to rely on "informal" healthcare providers (IHCPs). The level of formality in health provision is typically determined by a country's laws and regulations. IHCPs lack official qualifications required for providing health services (Bloom et al. 2011), are not registered with regulatory bodies, accept cash payments, and have no professional affiliations (Sudhinaraset et al. 2013). They offer affordable services, sometimes even lower in cost than those of free clinics when indirect costs like travel are taken into consideration (Amin et al. 2003). IHCPs can play a vital role in developing countries' healthcare systems, particularly in countries where there simply are not enough qualified medical practitioners to meet the needs of the community (Khare et al. 2019). In some countries, IHCPs act as a complementary provider to the formal healthcare system (Muzyamba et al. 2017; Shaikh et al. 2014; Kidia et al. 2017). While there is no universally agreed-upon definition of informal healthcare or IHCPs, a systematic review by Sudhinaraset et al. (2013) outlined a set of criteria to inform a definition. While formal healthcare systems and stakeholders may generally prioritize qualified healthcare providers, it is important to consider the context, specific roles, and contributions of IHCPs within the healthcare landscape. Operating within the community, IHCPs are often sought due to their accessibility, affordability, and established trust within the community (Kumar et al. 2021; Walker et al. 2001). The trust they gain stems from their understanding of social structures, cultural practices, and the community's approach to seeking healthcare (Magidson et al. 2019). Across Southeast Asia, IHCPs account for 55% of healthcare providers in India (Prasada Rao et al. 2017) and nearly 100% of all healthcare providers in rural Bangladesh (Sudhinaraset et al. 2013). In sub-Saharan Africa, nearly 50% of all pregnant women opt for traditional birthing attendants as opposed to a hospital, and 40% of people in Uganda will seek the help of healers to treat diarrhea (Twebaze 2001). However, because of the generally weaker governance in developing countries, it is difficult to regulate IHCP activities, particularly because they most often operate out of rural and remote locations. Poorly enforced policies and regulations mean that IHCPs can easily accumulate and dispense medications such as antibiotics (Gautham et al. 2011); however, they may be more likely to store medications incorrectly, which can render them ineffective (Chuc et al. 2001). The disadvantages of relying on IHCPs combined with geographical distance, poverty, lack of knowledge, and limited access to healthcare services pose a clear challenge to developing countries (Velez and Auseon 2014). While acknowledging IHCPs' important role in developing countries, there is a need to design comprehensive strategies that address the barriers to access and improve the overall healthcare system.

6.6 Conclusion

In summary, the issue of access to and equity in healthcare is a major challenge for both developed and developing countries. Access to healthcare is influenced by social, economic, cultural, and political factors that differentially affect citizens. The significant inequalities that exist at both the individual and macro levels and between countries living with varying levels of development are ongoing. While technological advancements have expanded access to healthcare through the digital environment, inequalities of access persist. Various theories, models, and frameworks that have been identified to address the issue of inequitable access to healthcare have had some, although limited, impact. A more integrated, collaborative approach between policymakers and all healthcare stakeholders is required if these challenges are to be addressed.

6.7 Reflective Pause Point

1. Do you have any experience, either as a healthcare provider or patient, of issues that have limited equal access and equity to healthcare?
2. Reflecting on your experiences, how might the adoption of any of the strategies for change identified above increase equitable access to healthcare for yourself or others?
3. What role might you play in improving equity of access to healthcare for yourself or for others for whom you have responsibility?

References

American Medical Association (2020) AMA Telehealth Implementation Playbook. https://www.ama-assn.org/system/files/ama-telehealth-playbook.pdf

Amin AA, Marsh V, Noor AM et al (2003) The use of formal and informal curative services in the mangement of paediatric fevers in four districts in Keny. Trop Med Int Health 8(12):1143–1152

Andermann A (2016) Taking action on the social determinants of health in clinical practice: a framework for health professionals. Can Med Assoc J 188(17–18):E474–E483. https://doi.org/10.1503/cmaj.160177

Artiga S, Orgera K (2020) Communities of color at higher risk for health and economic challenges due to COVID-19. Kaiser Family Foundation. https://www.kff.org/coronavirus-covid-19/issue-brief/communities-of-color-at-higher-risk-for-health-and-economic-challenges-due-to-covid-19/

Bashshur RL, Shannon GW, Metzner CA (1971) Some ecological differentials in the use of medical services. Health Serv Res 6(1):61–75

Berchick ER, Barnett JC, Upton RD (2019) Health insurance coverage in the United States: 2018. U.S. Census Bureau

Bloom GSH, Lucas H, Bhuiya A et al (2011) Making health markets work better for poor people: the case of informal providers. Health Policy Plan 26:i45–i52. https://doi.org/10.1093/heapol/czr025

Boulton JG, Allen PM, Bowman C (2015) Embracing complexity: strategic perspectives for an Age of Turbulence. Oxford University Press

Braveman P, Gruskin S (2003) Defining equity in health. J Epidemiol Community Health 57(4):254–258. https://doi.org/10.1136/jech.57.4.254

Bright T, Kuper H (2018) A systematic review of access to general healthcare services for people with disabilities in low and middle income countries. Int J Environ Res Public Health 15(9):1879. https://doi.org/10.3390/ijerph15091879

Chuc NT, Larsson M, Falkenberg T et al (2001) Management of childhood acute respiratory infections at private pharmacies in Vietnam. Ann Pharmacother 35(10):1283–1288. https://doi.org/10.1345/aph.10313

Cousins S (2020) COVID-19 has "devastating" effect on women and girls. Lancet 396(10247):301–302. https://doi.org/10.1016/S0140-6736(20)31679-2

Culyer AJ, Wagstaff A (1993) Equity and equality in health and health care. J Health Econ 12(4):431–457. https://doi.org/10.1016/0167-6296(93)90004-X

Curtis E, Jones R, Tipene-Leach D et al (2019) Why cultural safety rather than cultural competency is required to achieve health equity: a literature review and recommended definition. Int J Equity Health 18:174. https://doi.org/10.1186/s12939-019-1082-3

Donabedian A (1966) Evaluating the quality of medical care. Milbank Q 83(4):691–729

Frenk J (1992) Primary care and reform oh health systems: a framework for the analysis of Latin American experiences. Health Serv Manag Res 5(1):32–43. https://doi.org/10.1177/095148489200500104

Fronstin P (2019) What does the future hold for the employment-based health benefits system? E. I. Brief

Garzón-Orjuela N, Samacá-Samacá DF, Luque Angulo SC et al (2020) An overview of reviews on strategies to reduce health inequalities. Int J Equity Health 19(1):192. https://doi.org/10.1186/s12939-020-01299-w

Gautham M, Binnendijk E, Koren R et al (2011) 'First we go to the small doctor': first contact for curative health care sought by rural communities in Andhra Pradesh & Orissa, India. Indian J Med Res 134:627–638. https://doi.org/10.4103/0971-5916.90987

Hartley S, Raphael J, Lovell K et al (2020) Effective nurse-patient relationships in mental health care: a systematic review of interventions to improve the therapeutic alliance. Int J Nurs Stud 102:103490. https://doi.org/10.1016/j.ijnurstu.2019.103490

HealthIT (n.d.) The ONC HealthIT Playbook. https://www.healthit.gov/playbook/electronic-health-records/

Javanparast S, Freeman T, Labonté R et al (2018) How institutional forces, ideas and actors shaped population health planning in Australian regional primary health care organisations. BMC Public Health 18:383. https://doi.org/10.1186/s12889-018-5273-4

Keisler-Starkey K, Bunch LN (2022) Health insurance coverage in the United States: 2021. https://www.census.gov/content/dam/Census/library/publications/2022/demo/p60-278.pdf

Khare S, Purohit M, Sharma M et al (2019) Antibiotic prescribing by informal healthcare providers for common illnesses: a repeated cross-sectional study in rural India. Antibiotics 8(3):139

Kidia K, Machando D, Mangezi W et al (2017) Mental health in Zimbabwe: a health systems analysis. Lancet Psychiatry 4(11):876–886. https://doi.org/10.1016/S2215-0366(17)30128-1

Kumar R, Stevenson L, Jobling J et al (2021) Health providers' and pregnant women's perspectives about smoking cessation support: a COM-B analysis of a global systematic review of qualitative studies. BMC Pregnancy Childbirth 21(1):550. https://doi.org/10.1186/s12884-021-03773-x

Levesque JF, Harris MF, Russel G (2013) Patient-centred access to health care: Conceptualising access at the interface of health systems and populations. Int J Equity Health 12(1):18. https://doi.org/10.1186/1475-9276-12-18

Magidson JF, Jack HE, Rengenauer KS et al (2019) Applying lessons from task sharing in global mental health to the opioid crisis. J Consult Clin Psychol 87(10):962–966. https://doi.org/10.1037/ccp0000434

Manandhar M, Hawkes S, Buse K et al (2018) Gender, health and the 2030 agenda for sustainable development. Bull World Health Organ 96(9):644–653. https://doi.org/10.2471/BLT.18.211607
Marmot M (2005) Social determinants of health inequalities. Lancet 365(9464):1099–1104. https://doi.org/10.1016/S0140-6736(05)71146-6
Marmot M (2020) Social determinants of health inequalities. Lancet 395(10217):13–14. https://doi.org/10.1016/S0140-6736(19)32506-1
Muzyamba C, Groot W, Tomini SM et al (2017) The usefulness of traditional birth attendants to women living with HIV in resource-poor settings: the case of Mfuwe, Zambia. Tropical. Medicine and Health 45(37):37. https://doi.org/10.1186/s41182-017-0076-3
Naimoli JF, Frymus DE, Wuliji T et al (2014) A Community Health Worker "logic model": towards a theory of enhanced performance in low- and middle-income countries. Hum Resour Health 12:56. https://doi.org/10.1186/1478-4491-12-56
National Indigenous Australian Agencies (2020) Closing the Gap Report. Commonwealth of Australia. https://ctgreport.niaa.gov.au/sites/default/files/pdf/closing-the-gap-report-2020.pdf
OECD (2019) OECD economics surveys: India. https://www.oecd.org/economy/surveys/India-2019-OECD-economic-survey-overview.pdf
Orach CG (2009) Health equity: challenges in low income countries. Afr Health Sci 9:S49–S51
Penchansky R, Thomas JW (1981) The concept of access: definition and relationship to consumer satisfaction. Med Care 19(2):127–140. https://doi.org/10.1097/00005650-198102000-00001
Prasada Rao U, Nallapu S, Rao S (2017) The rural medical practitioner of India. J Evol Med Dent Sci 6(74):5321–5323. https://doi.org/10.14260/Jemds/2017/1154
Rapport MJ, Furze J, Martin K et al (2014) Essential competencies in entry-level pediatric physical therapy education. Pediatr Phys Ther 26(1):7–18. https://doi.org/10.1097/PEP.0000000000000003
Rodrigues CB, Thomaz EBAF, Batista RFL et al (2023) Prenatal care and human rights: addressing the gap between medical and legal frameworks and the experience of women in Brazil. PLoS One 18(2):e0281581. https://doi.org/10.1371/journal.pone.0281581
Rosenstock IM, Strecher VJ, Becker MH (1988) Social learning theory and the Health Belief Model. Health Educ Q 15(2):175–83. https://doi.org/10.1177/109019818801500203
Russell G, Kunin M, Harris MF et al (2019) Improving access to primary healthcare for vulnerable populations in Australia and Canada: protocol for a mixed-method evaluation of six complex interventions. Br Med J 9:e027869. https://doi.org/10.1136/bmjopen-2018-027869
Sen A (1999) Development as freedom. Knopf
Shaikh BT, Khan S, Maab A et al (2014) Emerging role of traditional birth attendants in mountainous terrain: a qualitative exploratory study from Chitral Distinct, Pakistan. BMJ Open 4(11):e006238. https://doi.org/10.1136/bmjopen-2014-006238
Shannon GW, Bashshur RL (1982) Accessibility to medical care among urban American Indians in a large metropolitan area. Soc Sci Med 16(5):571–575. https://doi.org/10.1016/0277-9536(82)90310-0
Sudhinaraset M, Ingram M, Lofthouse HK et al (2013) What is the role of informal healthcare providers in developing countries? A systematic review. PLoS One 8(2):e54978. https://doi.org/10.1371/journal.pone.0054978
The Global Fund (2022) Results report: https://www.theglobalfund.org/media/12265/corporate_2022resultsreport_report_en.pdf
Twebaze D (2001) A literature review of care-seeking practices for major childhood illnesses in Uganda. https://pdf.usaid.gov/pdf_docs/Pnacq731.pdf
United Nations (1948) Universal Declaration of Human Rights. https://www.un.org/en/about-us/universal-declaration-of-human-rights
United Nations (2015) Transforming our world: The 2030 Agenda for Sustainable Development. https://sdgs.un.org/2030agenda
Velez MR, Auseon AJ (2014) Defining characteristics of early adopters of multimodality cardiovascular imaging. Echocardiography 31(7):802–808. https://doi.org/10.1111/echo.12472

Walker D, Muyinda H, Foster S et al (2001) The quality of care by private practitioners for sexually transmitted diseases in Uganda. Health Policy Plan 16(1):35–40. https://doi.org/10.1093/heapol/16.1.35

Waters HR (2000) Measuring equity in access to health care. J Health Econ 51(4):599–612. https://doi.org/10.1016/S0277-9536(00)00003-4

Whitehead M (1992) The concepts and principles of equity and health. Int J Health Serv 22(3):429–445. https://doi.org/10.2190/986L-LHQ6-2VTE-YRRN

WHO (1948) Constitution of the World Health Organization. World Health Organization. http://www.who.int/governance/eb/who_constitution_en.pdf

WHO (2010) Telemedicine: Opportunities and developments in member states: Report on the Second Global Survey on eHealth 2009. http://www.who.int/goe/publications/goe_telemedicine_2010.pdf

WHO (2017) World Bank and WHO: half the world lacks access to essential health services, 100 million still pushed into extreme poverty because of health expenses. World Health Organization https://www.who.int/news/item/13-12-2017-world-bank-and-who-half-the-world-lacks-access-to-essential-health-services-100-million-still-pushed-into-extreme-poverty-because-of-health-expenses

WHO (2019) Closing the gap in a generation: health equity through action on the social determinants of health. World health Organization https://iris.who.int/bitstream/handle/10665/43943/9789241563703_eng.pdf

WHO (2020) Life expectancy and healthy life expectancy. World Health Organization https://www.who.int/data/gho

WHO (2022) Global spending on health: rising to the pandemic's challenges. World Health Organization https://apps.who.int/iris/bitstream/handle/10665/365133/9789240064911-eng.pdf

WHO (2023) Global health workforce statistics database. World Health Organisation. Retrieved April 28 from https://www.who.int/data/gho/data/themes/topics/health-workforce

Woldemichael A, Takian A, Akbari et al. (2019) Availability and inequality in accessibility of health Centre-based primary healthcare in Ethiopia. PLoS One 14(3), e0213896. https://doi.org/10.1371/journal.pone.0213896

Part II
Dare to Care: A Holistic Ecosystem of Health and Healthcare in Complexity

Part II of this book takes up the challenge identified in Part I of the need to go beyond pure description of changes that have been attempted to advance collaboration between professions, professionals and patients through teams, partnerships and leadership change, to explore elements of a holistic ecosystem of health and healthcare. The first four chapters (Chaps. 7, 8, 9 and 10) explore the importance of collaboration and the implications for changes collaboration, in modes of cognition, methods of action to build relationships and action to promote more collaboration engaged leadership. Three ecologies are assembled that focus on the three agencies of health and healthcare: Principles and Purpose (P1); People in Place (P2); Practices and Processes (P3). Resources are designed to assist change to be enabled. Chapters 11 and 12 discuss the need to recognize the spiritual in health and healthcare for the holistic ecosystem to be inclusive of Indigenous people. This is explored through discussion of the influence of Ancient Indigenous Wisdoms on Indigenous health and healthcare. A re-imagining of a closer alignment between Complexity science and Ancient Indigenous Wisdoms is considered, however it is concluded that identification of the many additional challenges for the holistic ecosystem in acknowledging the importance of spirit in Indigenous thinking adds a level of complexity that requires deeper consideration.

Chapter 7
Collaboration in Health and Healthcare

Sandra Jones

Abstract The aim of this chapter is to identify the challenges of, and opportunities for, collaboration in health and healthcare. Collaboration is discussed from both a micro (team level) and a macro (collaborative partnership and leadership level). Examples of changes at both the micro and macro level are presented. This discussion is complemented by the use of reflective practice to identify the implications for each of the 3P agencies of health and healthcare: Principles and Purposes (P1); (People in Place P2); and Practices and Processes (P3).

7.1 Introduction

In urging the adoption of a primary healthcare (PHC) approach, the World Health Organization (WHO) urged the adoption of "a whole-of-society approach designed to effectively organize and strengthen national health systems to bring services for health and wellbeing closer to communities" (WHO https://www.who.int/health-topics/primary-health-care#tab=tab_1). PHC outlines a vision for healthcare built on three components: i) implementing integrated health services to meet people's health needs throughout their lives, ii) addressing the broader determinants of health through multisectoral policy and action, and iii) empowering individuals, families, and communities to take charge of their own health. This chapter focuses on the second of these components, achieved through collaboration to develop and implement multisectoral policy.

S. Jones (✉)
Business and Law College, RMIT University, Melbourne, VIC, Australia

S. Jones, D. Vindigni OAM (eds.), *Health and Healthcare in Complexity*,
https://doi.org/10.1007/978-981-96-0515-6_7

7.2 Theories of Collaboration

Collaboration has long been acknowledged as "an ubiquitous presence in our lives and…a constant feature of modern society" (Patel et al. 2012, p. 1). Collaboration has been advocated to underpin the integration of health professionals, patients, and organizations involved in improving health and healthcare. Despite proposals to increase collaboration, there is no single agreed definition, theory, method, or practice of, and no single mandate for, collaboration for health and healthcare. Sullivan (1998, p. 6), for example, focused on the generic relationship between collaboration and power-sharing, describing collaboration as:

> a dynamic, transforming process of creating a power sharing partnership for pervasive application in health care practice, education, research, and organizational settings for the purposeful attention to needs and problems in order to achieve likely successful outcomes.

Hudson (1998), on the other hand, described a process of collaboration rather than its purpose, and claimed that collaboration is simply contingent on good communication and coordination. Kinnaman and Bleich (2004) described a spectrum of collaborative partnerships as, at the one end, simply tolerating different views, to, at the other end, transcending inequalities in power, decision-making, professional boundaries, and hierarchies. In between these two extremes are elements of collaboration described as co-ordination and co-operation. Explaining collaborative partnerships within community healthcare centers, Sicotte et al. (2000) described collaboration as a means for collective action aimed at developing a common "spiritual" goal of harmony and trust. This has led to the conclusion of Morley and Cashell (2017, p. 208) that:

> for a concept so widely used in everyday language, there is a surprising lack of a clear understanding of what it is to collaborate, and of how best to support and improve the practice of collaborative working.

These differences in definition and theory are further demonstrated in the variety of approaches to implementing collaboration in practice.

7.3 Practices of Collaboration

7.3.1 Collaboration Within Organizations

At the organizational level, collaboration has been dominated by discussion of teams. In healthcare, teams have been described as developing and adapting shared mental models between team members (Edmondson 1999). They are depicted as enabling individual members to "exercise skills for coordinating, cooperating and sharing decision-making based on agreed content, processes and behaviours"

(Morley and Cashell 2017, p. 211). Collaboration in teams, it is argued, enables individual members to "exercise skills for coordinating, cooperating and sharing decision-making based on agreed content, processes and behaviours" (Morley and Cashell 2017, p. 211). Edmondson (1999) claimed that team collaboration develops psychosocial safety for interpersonal risk-taking and the construction of shared mental models between team members (Edmondson 1999). However, teams are also criticized for having a negative impact on individual workers' attitudes, motivation, and cognition and reducing their engagement in work and ability to reach work targets (De Brun and McAuliffe 2020; Waldman et al. 2003). Such diverse findings led Morley and Cashell (2017) to suggest that the practice of collaboration needs to focus beyond teams to a range of factors including:

1. The synergistic alliances through which contributions can be maximized.
2. The engagement of multiple people from diverse backgrounds who are encouraged to build relationships that are based on valuing and respecting others' viewpoints and that aim at a common goal, supported by agreed strategies to address disagreements by seeking alternative solutions.
3. The encouragement of dynamic relations in which power is shared, communication is transformative, and negotiations are based on trust and respect.

7.3.2 Collaborative Partnerships Between Organizations

Collaborative partnerships have been advocated for practice-based health disciplines and professions, grassroots community groups, and stakeholders in the public, private, and nonprofit sectors, as well as between providers and patients and their families (Morley and Cashell 2017; Roussos and Fawcett 2000). Valentijn et al. 2013 described the spectrum of possible practices for collaborative partnerships as a "rainbow." For example, the conceptual framework for collaborative healthcare for social sustainability developed by Maghsoudi et al. (2020) identified a spectrum of possible practices and processes that vary from, at one extreme, simply communicating and sharing information and knowledge to, at the other extreme, sharing responsibility and joint decision-making. The conceptual framework to enable collaborative healthcare and social services integration developed by Cheng and Catallo (2020) added the need to consider broad differences between internal and external environments, national governance systems, funding arrangements and models, and health and social care policies. Given these differences, what is interesting is the elements that are common to all proposals that include the need for:

1. An identified common purpose.
2. Recognition of the importance of context on the way people interact.
3. An agreement on a common structure (formal or informal) and decision-making process (top-down or bottom-up).

7.3.3 Collaborative Partnerships Between Countries

Given the challenges to collaboration within and between organizations, it is little wonder that collaborative partnerships between countries are also hampered by lack of consensus on practice. While there is consensus that collaborative partnerships between low-income and high- and middle-income countries can improve population health, equity, and national development (Hanney and Gonzalez-Block 2013),[1] there is little agreement on collaborative partnership practices.

Initially collaboration was seen as synonymous with capacity development as the means to assist emerging economies to foster systematic, integrated approaches. (Bolger 2000). The UN Sustainability Development Goals, for example, emphasized the ethical obligation to foster social justice and health equity (Gostin and Sridhar 2014). Capacity development was based on a theory of relationship building between individuals, organizations, and broader systems and institutions (Morgan 1998). Lusthaus et al. (1999) advocated a participatory process aimed at broad-based participation coupled with a locally driven agenda designed to build local capacity by fostering ongoing learning and adaptation. Action to achieve such participation was focused on practices such as:

1. Raising awareness among global actors, funders, institutions, researchers, and ethical review boards.
2. Adopting a collectivist approach.
3. Establishing agreements between collaborating partners that ensure that reciprocal interests are protected and shared responsibilities and rewards recognized.
4. Facilitating communication and allocating resources, responsibilities, and project ownership among the parties (Ward et al. 2018).

In summary, while collaboration in health and healthcare has been broadly advocated, there is little agreement on the purpose of, or means, to achieve it. This suggests the need led to consider a form of leadership to encourage collaboration.

7.4 Leadership for Collaboration

Governments in several Western countries (notably Canada, the UK, and Australia) have encouraged multisectoral policy and action to support collaboration for public healthcare through the adoption of Distributed Leadership. While the specific aim in each case has differed, they share the underlying principle that, given the complex environment in which it is situated, the provision of healthcare service needs to be shared by multiple individuals (Leach et al. 2021).

In Canada in 2002, the Royal Commission on the Future of Health Care flagged the need for stronger leadership to sustain universal, prepaid hospital and medical

[1] See Chap. 6.

insurance programs through coalitions (Dickson and Tholl 2014). A national Canadian Health Leaders Network was established, based on a spirit of "leadership without ownership," with the aim being "to establish that leadership in health is everybody's business…within our sphere of influence…[in which] no one organization or profession owns leadership" (Dickson and Tholl 2014, p. viii). The Canadian LEADS framework, consisted of five action domains (Lead self; Engage others; Achieve results; Develop coalitions; and Transform systems) that was designed as a transformational, interactive, process-based form of distributed leadership (Dickson and Tholl 2014). It was built on several assumptions:

> the collective capacity of an individual or group to influence people to work together to achieve a common constructive purpose: the health and wellness of the population we serve…leadership as a process, not a position…. In health care, it could be from patients, providers at every level, politicians, or the public. What makes a person a leader is the ability to combine a commitment to improve with the knowledge of how to exercise influence and engage support. (Dickson and Tholl 2014, p. 2)

> That better leaders and better leadership go together, but they are not the same thing…so a leadership framework must be adaptable to different situations and responsive to the uniqueness of your needs. It also must allow for customization to reflect the unique qualities that distinguish us as individuals…by act[ing] as a common language for leadership. (Dickson and Tholl 2014, pp. 3–4)

In the UK, Distributed Leadership was adopted by the government in 2011 for health and social care. This was supported through the Kings Fund (2011) and incorporated into the National Health Service (NHS) leadership framework (NHS 2011). It was introduced in response to disillusionment about the ability of 'heroic models' of individual (role) leadership to address "wicked issues" (Currie and Lockett 2011). Distributed Leadership was identified as offering "a potential solution…by…enabling followers to take on leadership" (Currie and Lockett 2011, p. 287). In the UK case, a close link to adaptive leadership was identified through the adoption of shared principles and learning new ways that changed the focus from individuals to the collective: "instead of looking for saviours…[it enacted] leadership that will challenge us to face problems for which there is no simple, painless solution – problems that require us to learn new ways" (Heifetz 1994, p. 2). Distributed Leadership was considered to have the potential to encourage inclusivity, align with flatter organizational structures, foster collaboration and ethical practice, avoid alienation associated with lack of power, and encourage the application of skills and strengths across organizations, and thus enhance organizational effectiveness. Research undertaken within six years of the initial implementation in healthcare found evidence that a distributed leadership approach had contributed to the effectiveness of service delivery. Staff were identified as willing to share insights and accept responsibility for work adjustments, while health organizations and regional authorities adopted more strategic, interventionist approaches through devolution of authority to clinics (Beirne 2017). However, implementation faced a major institutional challenge of "internecine conflict between professions" (Currie and Lockett 2011, p. 294). This resulted in claims that clinicians without formal leadership titles were making "independent decisions regularly, inspiring change and driving improvements informally and collectively as front-line units or teams" (Beirne 2017, p. 8).

Australia adapted the Canadian LEADS framework in 2012 to create its first national health leadership framework. The Australian Health LEADS adopted the principle of leadership that would support a people-focused health system that was equitable, effective, and sustainable (Health Workforce Australia 2012). As in Canada, health networks were established to "bring together and recombine ideas and concepts from diverse domains" (Shannon and Sebastian 2017, p. 420). The Australian Health LEADS replaced the traditional problem-solving approach to leadership with a capacity-building approach that was guided by the belief that everyone owns, and shares responsibility for, leadership that is equitable, effective, and sustainable (Health Workforce Australia 2012). However, the Australian Health LEADS differed from the Canadian LEADS in three aspects. First, it adopted a more transactional approach between individuals in positions of leadership. Second, it focused on developing the capabilities of individual leaders. Third, it was less inclusive (Sebastian et al. 2014), focused on physicians rather than the broader range of healthcare stakeholders. Some expansion beyond the initial exclusive engagement of physicians did emerge over time with the engagement of a more diverse range of participants, but this was limited (Shannon and Sebastian 2017, p. 421). Further, when the Australian LEADS project was incorporated into the overall healthcare system, its impact declined.

In summary, while macro government level support for Distributed Leadership for healthcare did result in some change, it did not lead to sustainable collaboration at the micro level.

7.5 Discussion

The study of the literature on collaboration in health and healthcare has highlighted the need for further research into what constitutes collaboration and what is the relationship between collaboration and leadership. To create a basis upon which this research may be undertaken, the editors undertook reflection on the implications of the proposals for change discussed above for the 3P agencies of health and healthcare: Principles and Purposes (P1); People in Place (P2); and Practices and Processes (P3). The findings (Table 7.1) reveal the need for future research to achieve the following:

1. Parties agreeing on a common purpose/shared philosophy of collaboration and a more activity based approach to leadership.
2. Encouragement for multiple people from diverse background to engage in leadership by raising awareness and interest.
3. Establishment of practices and processes that flatten structures complemented by systems that encourage dynamic participation and shared decision-making.

Table 7.1 The 3P Agencies of Health and Healthcare: mapping the implications of proposals for change to encourage collaboration

3P agencies of health and healthcare	Collaboration within organizations	Collaboration (partnership) between organizations	Collaboration (partnerships) between countries	Distributed leadership
P1 Principles and Purposes	Form synergistic alliances to maximize contributions.	Identify a common purpose.	Form agreements that ensure focus on social justice, access, and health equity, and protect reciprocal interests.	Encourage inclusivity in which leadership is a process that is everybody's business.
P2 People and Place	Engage multiple people from diverse backgrounds in achieving a common goal.	Recognize the importance of context (environment) on the way people interact.	Foster a collectivist approach and focus on raising awareness.	Self-lead and engage others within context.
P3 Practices and Processes	Encourage dynamic relationships in which communication is transformative, negotiations are based in trust and respect, and power is shared.	Agree on a common structure and decision-making process.	Implement processes and communication to ensure shared funding, responsibilities, rewards, and project ownership.	Flatten organizational structures, develop a system-transformation focus on achieving results and developing capabilities, and make use of skills to build on strengths.

7.6 Conclusion

In summary, while the advantages of a more collaborative approach for health and healthcare are acknowledged, there is little agreement on either a single theory, model or practice of collaboration that has been proven to be successful and sustainable. While adopting Distributed Leadership for health and healthcare was aimed at engaging more people at the macro level, there is little evidence that it has led to significant micro level collaboration between professions and sub professions or between professionals and patients. Further research is needed to focus on changes needed.

7.7 Reflective Pause Point

1. Reflecting on your experience in healthcare workplaces, what opportunities have you had to engage in collaboration with other professions or with patients?
2. How would you describe the approach to leadership in your organization?
3. What actions are needed to further support collaboration in your workplace?

References

Beirne M (2017) The reforming appeal of distributed leadership. Br J Healthcare Manag 23(6):262–270. https://doi.org/10.1186/s12913-019-3883-x

Bolger J (2000) Why what and how of capacity development. Capacity Development Occasional Series 1(1):1–8. Canadian International Development Agency (CIDA) Policy Branch

Cheng S, Catallo C (2020) Conceptual framework; factors enabling collaborative healthcare and social services integration. J Integr Care 28(3):215–229

Currie G, Lockett A (2011) Distributed leadership in health and social care: concertive, conjoint or collective. Int J Manag Rev 13:286–300. https://doi.org/10.1111/j.1468-2370.2011.00308.x

De Brún A, McAuliffe E (2020) Identifying the context, mechanisms and outcomes underlying collective leadership in teams: building a realist programme theory. BMC Health Services Research, 20:1–13.

Dickson G, Tholl B (2014) Bringing leadership to life in health: leads in a caring environment a new perspective. Springer-Verlag, London

Edmondson AC (1999) Psychological safety and learning behavior in work teams. Adm Sci Q 44(2):350–383

Gostin LO, Sridhar D (2014) Global health and the law. N Engl J Med 370(18):1732–1740

Hanney SR, Gonzalez-Block MA (2013) Organising health research systems as a key to improving health: the world health report 2013 and how to make further progress. Health Res Policy Sys 11:47

Health Workforce Australia (2012) Health LEADS Australia: The Australian Health Leadership Framework. Retrieved from https://www.aims.org.au/documents/item/352

Heifetz R (1994) Leadership without easy answers. Harvard University Press, Cambridge, MA

Hudson B (1998) Prospects of partnership. Health Serv J 108:26–27

King's Fund (2011) The future of leadership and management in the NHS: no more heroes. Available at: http://www.kingsfund.org.uk/publications/future-leadership-and-management-nhs. Accessed 12 Sept 2022

Kinnaman M, Bleich M (2004) Collaboration: aligning resources to create and sustain partnerships. J Prof Nurs 20:310–322

Leach L et al (2021) Distributed leadership in healthcare: leadership dyads and the promise of improved hospital outcomes. Leadership in Health Services, 34(4):353–374.

Lusthaus C, Adrien MH, Pertinger M (1999) Capacity development; definitions, issues and implications for planning, monitoring and evaluation. Universalia Occasional Paper 35

Maghsoudi T, Cascón-Pereira R, Beatriz Hernández Lara A (2020) The role of collaborative healthcare in improving social sustainability: a conceptual framework. Sustain For 12(8):3195. https://doi.org/10.3390/su12083195

Morgan P (1998) Capacity and capacity development-some strategies'. Note prepared for the Political and Social Policy Division, Policy Branch, CIDA

Morley L, Cashell A (2017) Collaboration in health care. Journal of Medical Imaging and Radiation Sciences 48:207–216

NHS Institute for Innovation and Improvement (2011) NHS leadership framework: a summary. NHS, Coventry

Patel H, Pettit M, Wilson J (2012) Factors of collaborative working: a framework for a collaboration model. Appl Ergon 43:11–26

Roussos S, Fawcett S (2000) A review of collaborative partnerships as a strategy for improving community health. Annu Rev Public Health 21:369–402

Sebastian A, Fulop L, Dadich A et al (2014) Health LEADS Australia and implications for medical leadership. Leadersh Health Serv 27(4):355–370

Shannon S, Sebastian A (2017) Developing health leadership with Health LEADS Australia. Leadersh Health Serv 31(4):413–425

Sicotte C, D'Amour D, Moreault M (2000) Interdisciplinary collaboration within Quebec community health care centres. Soc Sci Med 55:991–1003

Sullivan T (1998) Collaboration: a health care imperative. McGraw-Hill, New York

Valentijn PP, Schepman SM, Opheij W et al (2013) Understanding integrated care: a comprehensive conceptual framework based on the integrative functions of primary care. Int J Integr Care 13(1):e010. https://doi.org/10.5334/ijic.886

Waldman HL et al (2003) Corporate culture of medicine hospital topics. Corporate culture: the missing piece of the healthcare puzzle 81(1): 5–14

Ward C-L, Shaw D, Sprumont D et al (2018) Good collaborative practice: reforming capacity building governance of international health research partnerships. Glob Health 14:1. https://doi.org/10.1186/s12992-017-0319-4

Chapter 8
Holistic Ecosystem of Health and Healthcare: Embracing Change in Cognition

Sandra Jones

Abstract The aim of this chapter is to discuss and reflect upon changes in modes of cognition designed to encourage collaboration that are aligned with principles of Complexity science for a holistic ecosystem of health and healthcare. It first discusses four modes of cognition: systems thinking, sensemaking, reflective thinking, and social ecological thinking. It then analyzes the implications of these modes of cognition for the three agencies of health and healthcare: Principles and Purposes (P1), People in Place (P2), and Practices and Processes (P3). The outcome is the assemblage of an ecology of cognition, termed the Collaborative Adaptive Resilient Ecology (CARE) of cognition for health and healthcare that is designed to encourage collaboration, adaptation, and relationships.

8.1 Complexity Science and Theory

Complexity is explained by Boulton, Allen, and Bowman (2015, p. 1) as a view of the world as:

> essentially interconnected, and rich with forms and patterns that have been shaped by history and context…[it] reminds us of the limits to certainty, it emphasizes that things are in a continual process of 'becoming' and that there is potential for startlingly new futures where what emerges can be unexpected and astonishing.

The complexity worldview is sandwiched between the mechanical and chaotic views of the world. In the mechanical:

> the world works like a machine…[in which] the future is a predetermined path inexorably unfolding from the present….we can analyse the facts, predict the future, decide how to intervene, make and execute plan, and control and measure outcomes. The world can be understood by breaking it down into constituent parts, and these can be dealt with in a piecemeal fashion. There is no learning, variety, adaptation, innovation or surprise. (Boulton et al. 2015, p. 1)

S. Jones (✉)
Business and Law College, RMIT University, Melbourne, VIC, Australia

S. Jones, D. Vindigni OAM (eds.), *Health and Healthcare in Complexity*,
https://doi.org/10.1007/978-981-96-0515-6_8

This is in contrast to the chaotic view of the world in which everything is unpredictable and without structure. In between these two extremes, Complexity science is the study of relations and interconnections between multiple disciplines as systems (Adner 2022; Pype et al. 2018; Davidson 2010; Begun et al. 2003). Complexity theory has been described as:

> the way forms, patterns, and institutions emerge and become established and are then constantly challenged and potentially invaded by the particular events, variations, decisions, shocks and so on that take place in particular places at particular times. (Boulton et al. 2015, p. 29)

The application of complexity thinking thus involves shifting focus to the whole to "learn how to think in terms of relationships, in terms of interconnections, patterns and context" (Boulton et al. 2015, p. 3). It involves consideration of systems that maintain their existence through the mutual interaction of their components. Battle-Fisher (2015, p. 1) described systems as:

> interconnecting parts that affect the integrity of the whole when the components change over time…[in which] systems denote interaction and flow of elements…[and is discoverable] through various systems approaches and methodologies. (Battle-Fisher 2015, p. 1)

Accordingly, a complex system differs from a traditional relationship that assumes a single, linear cause and effect association between two isolated events (Sweeney and Griffiths 2002), characterized as:

> self-organizing, adaptive, emergent, comprised of a large number of elements, autopoietic, nonlinear, dynamic, network-like in structure, open-ended with fuzzy boundaries, interdependent, agent-based, evolving, chaotic, comprised of feedback loops, historical, nodes within a larger network of systems, environmentally impacted, etc..... Together and in isolation, the characteristics of a complex system not only describe what it is; they explain how it works. (Castellani et al. 2015, p. 3)

In summary, while adoption of a complexity worldview is important, it is by its nature, complex to understand, explain, and implement. This is one of the reasons the mechanistic view has remained a dominant paradigm.

8.2 Health and Healthcare in Complexity

Studies of the implications of Complexity science for health and healthcare have highlighted the importance of interactions, relationships, the ability to self-organize, and diversity. McDaniel et al. (2013, p. 21) stated that healthcare is a "process of delivering services through complex adaptive systems with professionals and other knowledge workers as key participants in the direct delivery of care." In other words, a complex system is made up of:

> many interacting elements (agents) that coevolve with their local environment and they typically display the features of self-organization and emergent properties…that recognise the spontaneous emergence of order, structure, or stability in a system of many elements interacting only locally. (McDaniel et al. 2013, p. 7)

Pype et al. (2018) identified seven elements of collaboration within a distributed palliative home-care team functioning as a Complex Adaptive System (CAS);

1. A shared focus together with acknowledgement of the importance of negotiated agreements on sharing tasks and responsibilities.
2. Nonlinear interactions.
3. Mutual trust in and respect of each other's knowledge and expertise.
4. Good communications.
5. Interactions between team members that generate new behaviors and learning, skills acquisition, new ways of functioning, and new communication strategies.
6. Positive external factors, such as interprofessional collaboration training of new graduates and the reduction of the gap between public and private funding.
7. Positive interprofessional relationships that shape team effectiveness.

Despite recognition that health and healthcare need a new paradigm to function effectively in complexity, there has been little concerted effort to change. Boulton, Allen, and Bowman (2015, p. 5–6) claimed that the adoption of new methods, or ways of knowing and ways of acting, requires:

> *principles* and *frameworks* rather than step-by-step formulaic processes.... maxims and questions for consideration rather than rules....be[ing] wary of assuming everything can be tested and evidenced and imagine[ing] that we can always know what caused what or what might happen next.

This suggests that more attention needs to be given to developing a new ecology of cognition for the three agencies of health and healthcare: Principle and Purpose (P1), People in Place, and Practices and Processes (P3). To achieve this requires consideration of modes of cognition.

8.3 A New Paradigm of Cognition for Health and Healthcare[1]

Acknowledging complexity requires the adoption of a new paradigm consisting of new modes of thinking. The modes chosen for discussion in this chapter are systems thinking, sensemaking, reflective thinking, and social ecological thinking as discussed below.[2]

---

[1] The next chapter will discuss operational and relationship changes, while the following chapter will discuss changes to leadership.

[2] The author acknowledges there may be other maxims and questions for consideration but maintains that these serve as an effective place to start.

8.3.1 Systems Thinking

Adoption of Complexity science has been accompanied by the replacement of linear (or analytical) thinking with systems thinking (Capra 1996, p. 30). Systems thinking incorporates an understanding and recognition that:

1. The organization of the whole can only be seen from an understanding of the parts "whose essential properties arise from the relationships between its parts" (Capra 1996, p. 27). It is upon these that effective systems-based practice is based through the identification and understanding of the interrelationships between the parts of the complex whole (Batalden and Moor 1997; Bowe and Armstrong 2017).
2. Nonlinearity exists between cause and effect (Khan et al. 2018, p. 1).
3. Social elements are often unpredictable and uncontrollable (Battle-Fisher 2015).
4. There is a constant interplay of elements (Battle-Fisher 2015), with relationships between elements being complex and open-ended and often not reliant on rules, but still assuming a prevalence of order (Snowden and Standbridge 2004).
5. There is an overarching link between the five principles of learning (personal mastery, mental models, building shared visions, team learning, and systems thinking), (Senge 1990).

Systems thinking is concerned with identifying interconnections as a key element of a broader and more holistic worldview that, in fact, may accelerate change (Evitts et al. 2010). Systems thinking is used to identify emerging stable patterns, although it is also recognized that in practice they may 'wobble' or fluctuate because they are made up of a collection of individual and varied actions and behaviors (Boulton et al. 2015, p. 29). This means that while systems analysis is "helpful in describing stability, they tell us little about change, what may cause it and what may emerge as a result" (Boulton et al. 2015, p. 31).

Despite these limitations, systems thinking enables a focus on the detail that contributes to a holistic perspective in which health and healthcare can be in "a balanced dynamic state between one's physical and emotional experiences, one's social connectedness, and most importantly one's sensemaking abilities-defining a somato-psycho-socio-semiotic (SPSS) model of health" (Sturmberg 2022, p. 2). Systems thinking enables recognition and consideration of the many microsystems that are interdependent, hierarchical, and embedded and that occur at multiple (micro, meso, and macro) levels (Begun et al. 2003).

However, a limitation is that systems thinking assumes the prevalence of order that is uncharacteristic of the messy and unpredictable nature of contemporary health systems. Accordingly, for systems thinking to assist a paradigm change in modes of cognition in health and healthcare, there is need to add sensemaking that helps identify and understand emerging patterns (Belrhiti et al. 2018).

8.3.2 Sensemaking

Sensemaking provides agents with the opportunity to operate effectively in both ordered and unordered situations. While systems thinking assists in the identification of the diverse agencies involved in health and healthcare (delivery providers, patients, and funding bodies) (Gulick 2019), sensemaking identifies the interrelationships between these agencies. Weick et al. (2005, pp. 409–410) described sensemaking as:

(i) A process that enables "circumstances to be turned into a situation…that is comprehended explicitly in words and that serves as a springboard into action".
(ii) Enabling exploration of "the interplay of action and interpretation rather than the influence of evaluation on choice…[that involves] the ongoing retrospective development of plausible images that rationalise what people are doing".
(iii) Capturing "the realities of agency, flow equivocality, transience, re-accomplishment, unfolding, and emergence, realities that are often obscured by the language of variables, nouns, quantities and structures".

In essence, sensemaking adds a process of collaboration through reciprocal exchanges between actors (enactment) and their environment (ecological change) that enables meaningful (selection) and preservation (retention). Through sensemaking people are able to "mak*[e]* sense of inputs and enact*[ing]* the sense back into the world to provide some order to move out of chaos" (Weick et al. 2005, p. 410).

In combination, systems thinking and sensemaking provide the means to respond to the uncertainty of health and healthcare by "engaging diverse individuals that create a process by which, as individuals interact, dynamically, stable patterns of organizing develop over time" (Lanham et al. 2020, p. 127). It has been applied in healthcare to:

(i) Identify collaboration between interprofessional patient-partnered care teams for clinical diagnosis of patients, "the group interacts in caring for patients, they exchange and process information, learn, and adapt their behaviour over time" (Lanham et al. 2020, p. 127).
(ii) Replace a single focus on human action with a focus on performativity of practice "through which certain ways of acting became enacted as sensible" (Hultin and Mahring 2017, p. 566).
(iii) Identify patterns of behavior that emerge during uncertainty (Rutledge 2009).
(iv) Lead to more open communication in situations with a high degree of ambiguity, uncertainty, disorder, or chaos by enabling willing participants to use retrospection to make sense of observed puzzles as they experience specific uncertainties and as they start to ask what has happened and is happening that is affecting their work (Lanham et al. 2020).

Rutledge (2009) outlined a four step process for sensemaking that:

(i) Commences with asking a question (what is this about?).

(ii) Proceeds to identify action needed to extract, label, and categorize clues aimed at stabilizing the streaming of experience through answering bracketed concerns or question(s) and presents the opportunity for plausibility to gain precedence over accuracy as participants create new understanding through approximations or plausible images.
(iii) Identifies actions and creates a path to move along based on questions of what's going on in a given situation and leads to a question of what participants should do next.
(iv) Concludes with ongoing refinement as new patterns emerge. In this latter stage, sensemaking is assisted by reflective thinking.

8.3.3 Reflective Thinking

Reflection has been described as:

> a process of thinking, feeling, imagining and learning by considering what has happened in the past, what might be happening if things had been done differently, what is currently happening and what could possibly happen in the future. (Rolfe 2011, p. 13)

Building on Dewey's (1938) early model of reflective thinking as the construction of knowledge through retrospective contemplation of practice, Gibbs (1988) identified a reflective framework based on three aspects of a situation:

1. Description of what happened.
2. Evaluation of the good and bad points and attempts to make sense of it.
3. Development of a conclusion and action plan as to what could have been done and what might be done in the future.

Reflective practice underpins the opportunity to connect and interconnect ways of thinking between individuals in a team or a whole of organization that can "transform experience into better and more actionable knowledge" (Ghaye and Lillyman 2010, p. 26):

> Traditionally, change and practice improvement were seen as a matter of human agency…more recently, increasing attention has been placed upon the organizational culture/s in which clinicians and those responsible for healthcare management are situated…this shifts our attention onto the interdependence between supportive and learning enriched clinical settings and practice that is safe and of high quality. (Ghaye and Lillyman 2010, p. 28)

Critical thinking adds the ability to address the criticism that reflection provides "no guidelines or cue questions to help practitioners to apply that knowledge back to practice beyond asking themselves to think about what they would do if the situation arose again" (Rolfe 2011, p. 36). Critical reflection enables transformation of the way practitioners view the world and their place in it to create and clarify "the meaning of experience in terms of self in relation to both self and the world" (Boyd and Fales 1983, p. 101). This has led critical reflection to be termed an emancipatory domain (Habermas 1974).

Three forms of reflective thinking have been applied to nursing and practices (Taylor 2006, p. 103). Technical reflection enables assessment of planning, implementing, and evaluating actions; Practical reflection enables a focus on experiencing, interpreting, and learning from experience; and Critical (emancipatory) reflection enables consideration of action to construct, deconstruct, confront, and reconstruct practices.

In combination, the three modes of cognition, systems thinking, sensemaking, and reflective thinking, can make a positive contribution to a holistic ecosystem of health and healthcare in complexity. It can replace the traditional 'deficit approach', with a 'strengths-based approach' that focuses on identifying, amplifying, and contextualizing successes (Ghaye and Lillyman 2010). It can assist the acknowledgement of the uniqueness of health and healthcare that makes it difficult to apply cost-benefit analysis, the need to acknowledge highly variable time horizons, and the nature of indeterminate technologies (McDaniel et al. 2013, p. 21).

While together these three modes provide building blocks for a change in cognition, consideration of how they may connect and interconnect requires consideration of a fourth mode of cognition, social ecological thinking.

8.3.4 Social Ecological Thinking

Ecological thinking enables consideration of broad change in:

> theories, disciplines, methods, practices and mandates…[to] simultaneously address issues of social justice, ecological integrity and social, physical and mental health and well-being. (Gislason and Bendelow 2013, p. xvi)

Ecological thinking has been used to explain the transformation of the energy in ecosystems as complex interactions between biological organisms, social beings, and the environment (Bubolz and Sontag 2009). The original conceptualization of ecosystems as holistic, dynamic interconnections between the natural world and human society (plants, microorganisms, and animals) has been expanded, initially into human ecological thinking, and thence into broader social and economic interconnections.

Expanding beyond its initial conceptualization, ecological thinking has been used as a metaphor for complex human activity to identify ecosystems of human development (Bronfenbrenner 1979; Bronfenbrenner and Ceci 1994), community psychology (Kelly et al. 2000), psychology of organizations as open systems (Katz and Kahn 1978), and social ecosystems that reflect the dynamics of public life and private enterprise such as in education and social care. It has also been applied to the wider world of governance and politics (Hodgson and Spours 2016; Hodgson and Spours 2013) and to business to go "beyond the binaries of marketization, on the one hand, and top-down managerialism, on the other hand" (Hodgson and Spours 2016, p. 36). In the case of health and healthcare, social ecological thinking presents the opportunity to shape and develop a different future from that of simply being an extension of the present.

In each of the above applications of ecological thinking, there is recognition of the presence of multiple reciprocal interactions between people, objects, and symbols (biological, psychological, and context). The human behavior ecosystem recognizes five levels of context that connect the individual through reciprocal interactions: first, to objects, symbols, and the biologically inherited factors of sex, age, and health; second, to the immediate (microsystem) environment that surrounds the individual; third, to the mesosystem; fourth, to the exosystem; fifth to the macrosystem; and, sixth to the chronosystem of society (Bronfenbrenner and Ceci 1994). Business ecosystems, such as Google and Apple, have identified four interrelated elements of self-sustaining business systems: a catalyst to trigger development, world-class research to provide a stream of new talent, a regulatory regime sympathetic to risk-taking and interdependence to attract and retain knowledge workers, and cooperation among actors through flatter hierarchies and strong networks (Finegold 1999). Social ecosystems have recognized connections and holistic thinking between various levels of human existence (the individual, families, communities, regions, societies, and nations) and the planet itself (Hodgson and Spours 2016).

Applied to health and healthcare, social ecological thinking has been used to inform medical ideologies and practices for disease prevention in public health and health-promotion programs (Gislason and Bendelow 2013; Roussos and Fawcett 2000; McLeroy et al. 1988; Stokols 1992) and as the means to identify an integrated approach to health (Kingsley and Thomas 2017). This has led to healthcare researchers being encouraged to:

> interrogate their underlying assumptions and beliefs, examine dominant narratives and question power structures that persist across field developments..[to go beyond].. simply gathering specialists to provide 'expert' opinion…to assess issues collectively from various perspective. (Buse et al. 2018, p. 422)

8.4 Discussion: An Ecology of Cognition for Health and Healthcare

To explore how these four modes of thinking may assist in developing a new ecology of cognition for health and healthcare, a four-phase reflection approach was undertaken by the editors.

In the first reflection phase, the four modes of thinking were examined for their genuineness and comprehensiveness in identifying changes required of the three agencies of health and healthcare: Principles and Purposes (P1); People in Place (P2); and Practices and Processes (P3). The findings, summarised in Table 8.1, are discussed below:

Table 8.1 The 3P Agencies of Health and Healthcare: mapping the implications of change in modes of cognition

3P agencies of health and healthcare	Systems thinking	Sensemaking	Reflective thinking	Social ecological thinking
P1 **Principles and Purposes** *Systems, relations, and interconnections*	Parts understood through the organization as a whole	Flows, unfolding, and emergence are captured	Enables a mix of technical and practical reflection	Recognises agencies in dynamic interconnections
P2 **People in Place** *Interacting agents—collaborate and coevolve through interactions, relationships, self-organization, and diversity*	Relationships between elements are seen as open-ended systems that assume the prevalence of order	Collaboration is achieved through interrelationships based on reciprocal exchange	Extend beyond the individual to the collective	Includes professionals, patients, families, and communities in accord with the context and culture
P3 **Practices and Processes** *Spontaneous emergence of order, structure, stability, and adaptability*	Interdependent microsystems are identified that are hierarchical and embedded and occur at multiple levels	Circumstances are turned into situations as a springboard to action	Enables the creation and clarification of meaning through the application of critical reflection	Enables collaboration for holistic and public health
Interactions through feedback loops, information sharing	Acknowledges nonlinearity	Decenters humans and foregrounds performativity of practice	Extends change and practice from an exclusive focus on human agency to organizational culture	Encourages integration between separated professions
Impact of external factors including training, finance, and public attitude	Harnesses understanding of unpredictable and uncontrollable social elements	Recognizes enactment, ecological change, selection, and retention	Encourages critical reflection on self in relation to both self and to the world	Encourages a mix of clinical (technical) and individual (lived) experiences
Knowledge growth and team behavior	Encourages open communication within a high degree of ambiguity, uncertainty, disorder, or chaos	Leads to identification of (plausible) new patterns	Leads to the construction of new knowledge through the retrospective contemplation of practice	Leads to shaping and development of a different future

8.4.1 Principles and Purposes (P1)

The first agency (P1) is identified as providing the means to ensure commitment to a common principle and purpose upon which collaboration can be built. Linking this to the four modes of thinking identifies the opportunity to: use systems thinking to help identify emerging patterns; sensemaking to capture flows of unfolding and emergent activity; reflective thinking to consider issues from a mix of technical and emotional perspectives; and social ecological thinking to identify dynamic interconnections between agencies.

8.4.2 People in Place (P2)

The second agency (P2) is identified as engaging people with diverse expertise in developing and co-evolving shared commitment to collaboration. This can be achieved through the employment of: systems thinking to provide the opportunity to identify relationships built as part of open-ended systems that assume an element of order; sensemaking that presents the opportunity to build collaboration through reciprocal exchange; reflective thinking that extends the focus beyond the individual to the collective; and social ecological thinking that assists recognition of the important contribution of individuals (professionals, patients, community) in accord with specific contexts and cultures.

8.4.3 Practices and Processes (S3)

The third agency (P3) is identified as designing the means to focus on internal systems, dynamic interactions and acknowledge external influences. This requires action to:

(i) Develop systems that support the spontaneous emergence of order, structure, stability, and adaptability. This to be achieved by utilizing: systems thinking to identify patterns between the multiple, interdependent microsystems at multiple levels; sensemaking to turn circumstances into situations that can springboard new action; reflective thinking to identify opportunities to create and clarify meaning; and social ecological thinking to focus on collaboration.

(ii) Create dynamic interactions with feedback loops for information sharing. This to be achieved by utilizing: systems thinking to provide the means to focus on nonlinearity; sensemaking to decenter human performativity and foreground performativity of practice; reflective thinking to extend change and practice beyond an exclusive focus on human agency and embrace organizational culture; and social ecological thinking to focus on integration.

(iii) Acknowledge external factors. This to be achieved by utilizing: systems thinking to recognize the impact of social elements on patterns that are often unpredictable and uncontrollable; sensemaking to recognize the enactment and social ecological exchange involved in selection and retention of the appropriate elements; reflective thinking to develop an awareness of self in relation to the external world; and social ecological thinking to focus on health and healthcare from both a clinical (technical) and an individual (lived) experience.

(iv) Implement systems and processes to develop shared understanding and to support for continuous growth in knowledge and in improved team behavior. This to be achieved by utilising: systems thinking to develop patterns of communication in situations in which there is a high degree of ambiguity, uncertainty, disorder, and chaos; sensemaking to identify plausible new patterns; reflective (critical) thinking to construct new knowledge through retrospective contemplation of practice and social ecological thinking to focus on developing different futures.

In the second reflection phase, the inter-relationship between these four modes of thinking was considered. This resulted in identification of a potential nested approach in which systems thinking provides the basis upon which sensemaking, reflective practice and social ecological thinking can establish links within, between and across each other. Applying sensemaking to systems thinking enables identification of emerging patterns; adding reflection thinking enables consideration of new actions based on lessons learnt from past practice; considering social ecological thinking enables interrogation of underlying assumptions.

In the third reflection phase consideration was given to how these inter-connected modes of thinking can be assembled into a holistic ecology of cognition to encourage collaboration, adaptation, and resilience in the face of variation. This is in accord with what Khan et al. (2018, p. 193) described as collaboration in which agencies "receive, learn and adapt to feedback to develop a shared value system that leads to the evolution and transformation of systems to facilitate adaptation." This resulted in the assemblage of an ecology of cognition, termed the *Collaborative Adaptive Resilient Ecology (CARE) of cognition* for health and healthcare illustrated in Fig. 8.1.

Having identified an ecology of cognition, the fourth reflection phase, aimed to create a resource to assist individuals and groups to design a program of action based on these modes of thinking and their interconnections. This resource, in the form of a Template, was designed to encourage understanding of how the CARE can be used to help implement a holistic ecology of health and healthcare. This reflection took into account the descriptors of the four modes of thinking for each of the 3Ps. It resulted in the design of a resource, consisting of 24 reflection prompts (formulated from the descriptors of the four modes of thinking) for the 3Ps to adapt as appropriate for different contexts and cultures. The resource is termed the *Self-Enabling Ecology of Reflection on Cognition* [Template 8.1 *SEER C*].

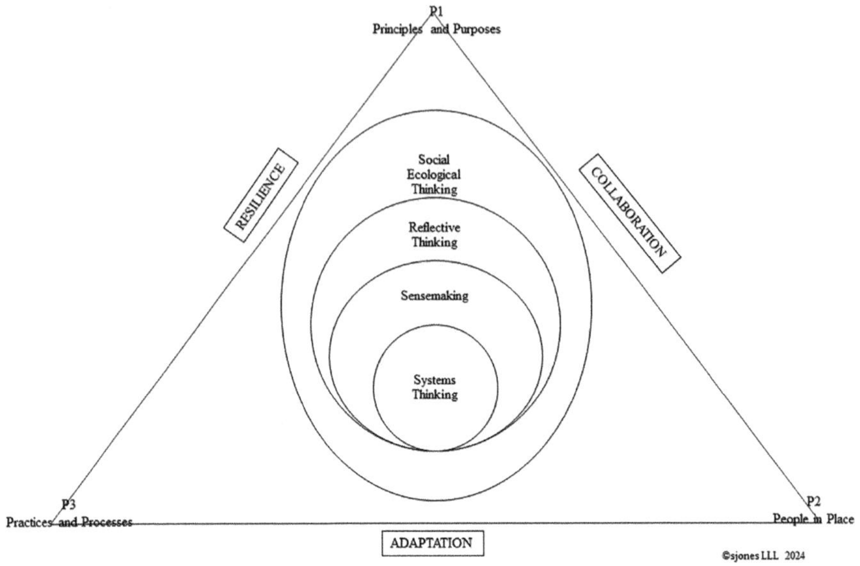

Fig. 8.1 A Collaborative Adaptive Resilient Ecology (CARE) of Cognition for Health and Healthcare

Template 8.1 Self-Enabling Ecology of Reflection on Cognition (SEER C)

Use the reflection prompts to identify changes in cognition associated with each of the modes of thinking…

3P agencies of health and healthcare	Systems thinking	Sensemaking	Reflective thinking	Social ecological thinking
P1 **Principles and purposes** *systems, relations and interconnections*	*…encourage understanding of the organisation as a whole*	*…encourage the unfolding and emergence of new systems*	*…focus on emergence of solutions based on lessons learnt*	*…encourage understanding of dynamic interconnections between all agencies*
P2 **People in place** *agents who collaborate and co-evolve through interactions, relationships, self-organisation and diversity*	*…enable relationships between elements to seek future order arising from complexity*	*…enact collaborative, reciprocal relationships*	*…encourage reflection beyond the individual to the collective*	*…engage professionals, patients, families and communities*
P3 **Practices and processes** *spontaneous emergence of order, structure, stability and adaptability*	*…enact interdependent microsystems that are embedded at multiple levels*	*…encourage circumstances to be turned into situations as springboards to action*	*…create and clarify meaning through critical reflection*	*…collaborate to achieve a holistic approach to public health*
interactions through feedback loops and information sharing	*…encourage non-linear thinking*	*…evaluate performativity of practice*	*…evaluate inclusive of human agency and culture*	*…encourage integration between separated professions*
external factors (training, finance, public attitude)	*…encourage "living with" unpredictable and uncontrollable elements*	*…encourage thinking based on ecological change*	*…critically reflect on self in relation to self, and to the world*	*…mix clinical (technical) and individual (lived) experience*
knowledge growth and team behaviour	*…encourage open communication in ambiguity, uncertainty, disorder or chaos*	*…focus on emergent patterns*	*…enable new knowledge through retrospective contemplation of practice*	*…encourage acceptance of emergence (rather than blame) to shape and develop futures*

8.5 Conclusion

This chapter locates health and healthcare within Complexity science to explore a paradigm shift in modes of cognition to assist the implementation of collaboration for a holistic ecosystem of health and healthcare. Four modes of cognition: systems thinking, sensemaking, reflective thinking, and social ecological thinking, were chosen for consideration. By employing a reflective practice approach, a *Collaborative Adaptive Resilient Ecology (CARE)* of cognition for health and healthcare, was assembled. To assist the use of the new paradigm of cognition to support the implementation of a holistic ecosystem of health and healthcare, a resource in the form of a template 8.1, termed a *Self-Enabling Ecology of Reflection on Cognition [SEER C],* as created. The SEER C is designed to be used by individuals and groups to self-identify how to use the four modes of thinking to achieve a paradigm change in cognition to support a holistic ecosystem of health and healthcare that is appropriate to specific contexts and cultures.

References

Adner R (2022) Sharing value for ecosystem success. MIT Sloan Management Review: 85–90

Batalden PB, Mohr JJ (1997) Building knowledge of health care as a system. Qual Manag Health Care 5(3):1–12

Battle-Fisher M (2015) Application of systems thinking to health policy & public health ethics, SpringerBriefs in Public Health. Springer. https://doi.org/10.1007/978-3-319-12203-8-1

Begun JW, Zimmerman B, Dooley KJ (2003) Health care organizations as complex adaptive systems. In: Mick SS, Wyttenbach ME (eds) Advances in health care organization theory. Jossey-Bass, San Francisco, pp 253–288

Belrhiti Z, Giralt A, Marchal B (2018) Complex leadership in healthcare: a scoping review. Int J Healthcare Manag 7(12):1073–1084

Boulton JG, Allen PM, Bowman C (2015) Embracing complexity: strategic perspectives for an Age of Turbulence. Oxford University Press

Bowe C, Armstrong A (2017) Assessment for systems learning: a holistic assessment framework to support decision making across the medical education continuum. Acad Med 92(5):585–592

Boyd E, Fales A (1983) Reflective learning: the key to learning from experimentation. J Humanst Psychol 23(2):99

Bronfenbrenner U (1979) The ecology of human development: experiments by nature and design. Harvard University Press, Cambridge

Bronfenbrenner U, Ceci SJ (1994) Nature-nurture reconceptualized in developmental perspective: A bioecological model. Psychol Rev 101(4):568–586

Bubolz MM, Sontag MS (2009) Human ecology theory. In: Boss P, Doherty WJ, LaRossa WR, Steinmetz SK (eds) Sourcebook of family theories and methods. Ch17. Springer, Boston MA, pp 419–450

Buse CG, Oestreicher JS, Ellis NR et al (2018) Public health guide to field developments linking ecosystems, environments and health in the Anthropocene. J Epidemiol Community Health 72:420–425

Capra F (1996) The web of life: a new synthesis of mind and matter. Harper Collins Publishers

Castellani B, Rajaram R, Buckwater J.G et al (2015) Place and Health as Compx Systems: A Case Study and Empirical test. Springer Briefs in Public Health. Springer International Publication:Switzerland. http://www.springer.com/series/10138.

Davidson SJ (2010) Complex responsive processes: a new lens of leadership in twenty-first century healthcare. Nurs Forum 45(2):108–117

Dewey J (1938) Experience and education. Macmillan, New York

Evitts S, Seale B, Skybrook D (2010) Supporting strategic sustainable development. In: Masters in strategic leadership toward sustainability thesis: interview questionnaire, Blenkinge Institute of Technology, Sweden

Finegold D (1999) Creating self-sustaining, high-skill ecosystems, Oxford review of 33. Econ Policy 15(1):60–81

Ghaye T, Lillyman S (2010) Reflection: principles and practices for healthcare professionals. Andrews UK Ltd

Gibbs G (1988) Learning by doing: a guide to teaching and learning methods. Oxford Polytechnic, Oxford, Further Education Unit

Gislason M, Bendelow G (2013) Introduction. In: Gislason M (ed) Ecological health: society, ecology and health. Emerald Publishing Limited

Gulick PG Jr (2019) A systems thinking approach to health care reform in the United States, 21 DePaul J. Health Care L. Available at: https://via.library.depaul.edu/jhcl/vol21/iss1/1

Habermas J (1974) Theory and practice. Heinemann, London

Hodgson A, Spours K (2013) An ecological analysis of the dynamics of localities: a 14+ low opportunity progression equilibrium in action. J Educ Work 28(1):24–43

Hodgson A, Spours K (2016) The evolution of social ecosystem thinking: its relevance for education, economic development and localities. A Stimulus paper for the UCL Ecosystem Seminar Organised by the Centre for Post-14 Education and Work, UCL Institute of Education, Accessed 25 Nov 2022 through discovery.ucl.ac.uk

Hultin L, Mahring M (2017) How practice makes sense in healthcare operations: studying sense-making as performative, material-discursive practice. Hum Relat 70(5):566–593

Katz D, Kahn RL (1978) The social psychology of organizations, 2nd edn. John Wiley and Sons, New York

Kelly JG, Ryan AM, Altmann BE et al (2000) Understanding and changing social systems: an ecological view. In: Rappaport J, Seidman E (eds) Handbook of community psychology. Plenum, New York, pp 133–159

Khan S, Vandermorris A, Shepherd J et al (2018) Embracing uncertainty, managing complexity: applying complexity thinking principles to transformation efforts in healthcare systems. BMC Health Serv Res 18:192. https://doi.org/10.1186/s12913-018-2994-

Kingsley J, Thomas S (2017) Ecosystem approaches to community health and wellbeing: towards an integrated Australian governance framework in response to global environmental change. EcoHealth 14:210–213. https://doi.org/10.1007/s10393-016-1193-x

Lanham H, Pugh J, Aron D et al (2020) Sensemaking as a strategy for managing uncertainty. In: Rapport F, Braithwaite J (eds) Transforming healthcare with qualitative research. Taylor & Francis Group. ProQuest Ebook Central. http://ebookcentral.proquest.com/lib/rmit/detail.action?docID=6355256. Created from rmit on 2022-09-29 12:28:02

McDaniel RR, Driebe DJ, Lanham H (2013) Health care organizations as complex systems: new perspectives on design and management. In: Friedman L (ed) Annual Review of Health Care Management: Revisiting the Evolution of Health Systems Organization. Emerald Publishing Limited, pp 3–26. ProQuest Ebook Central, http://ebookcentral.proquest.com/lib/rmit/detail.action?docID=1602362. Created from rmit on 2023-06-15 01:15:58

McLeroy BD, Steckler A, Glanz K (1988) An ecological perspective on health promotion programs. Health Edu Qual 15:351–377

Pype P, Mertens F, Helwaut F et al (2018) Healthcare teams as complex adaptive systems: understanding team behaviour through team members' perception of interpersonal interaction. BMC Health Serv Res 18(1):570. https://doi.org/10.1186/s12913-018-3392-3

Rolfe G (2011) Knowledge and practice. In: Rolfe J, Jasper M, Freshwater D (eds) Critical reflection in practice, Ch, vol 2, 2nd edn. Palgrave Macmillan, Basingstoke, Hampshire, pp 11–29
Roussos S, Fawcett S (2000) A review of collaborative partnerships as a strategy for improving community health. Annu Rev Public Health 21:369–402
Rutledge M (2009) Sensemaking as a tool in working with complexity, OD. Practitioners 41(2):19–24
Senge PM (1990) The art and practice of the learning organization. Currency Doubleday, New York
Snowden D, Standbridge P (2004) The landscape of management: creating the context for understanding social complexity. Emerg: Complex Organ 6(1–2):140–148
Sturmberg J (2022) There is more to 'making connections to improve health outcomes'. Glob Adv Health Med 11:1–3
Sweeney K, Griffiths F (2002) Complexity and healthcare: an introduction. Radcliffe Medical Press Ltd, Oxon
Taylor B (2006) Reflective practice: a guide for nurses and midwives, 2nd edn. Open University Press, Buckingham
Weick K, Sutcliffe K, Obstfeld D (2005) Organizing and the process of sensemaking. Organ Sci 16(4):409–421

Chapter 9
Holistic Ecosystem of Health and Healthcare: Actioning Change to Build Relationships

Sandra Jones

Abstract The aim of this chapter is to discuss and reflect upon four methods of action designed to build relationships for collaboration that are aligned with the principles of Complexity science applied to a holistic ecosystem of health and healthcare. It first discusses the four methods of action to build relationships: distributive engagement, networking, participatory action research, and reflexive practice. It then analyzes the implications of these methods for the three agencies of health and healthcare: Principles and Purposes (P1); People in Place (P2); and Processes and Practices (P3). The outcome is the assemblage of an ecology of action to build relationships, termed the Distributive Action Relational Ecology (DARE) of health and healthcare. Finally, it reflects upon the link between modes of cognition (identified in the Chap. 8) and actions to build relationships. The Chapter concludes with the assemblage of an ecology of cognition and action, termed the DARE to CARE for health and healthcare.

9.1 Open, Dynamic, Interconnected System

The complex world is systemic and cannot be understood without exploring interconnections beyond linear assumptions that make problems complicated. Boulton et al. (2015) argued that in a complex world, interconnections need to be identified by looking widely, seeking patterns of connections, and making assumptions that knowledge is held in the forms that emerge from the resulting interdependencies and reflexive connections. Complexity theory assumes open systems "where energy and information are exchanged with the wider world and the importance of the unique details of events and individual characteristics which are not

S. Jones (✉)
Business and Law College, RMIT University, Melbourne, VIC, Australia

S. Jones, D. Vindigni OAM (eds.), *Health and Healthcare in Complexity*,
https://doi.org/10.1007/978-981-96-0515-6_9

amenable to translation into deterministic mathematical equations" (Boulton et al. 2015, p. 33). The outcome is that complex systems are ambiguous, diffuse, and evolutionary and consist of many things that overlap and interact and cannot be easily modeled or measured. Boulton et al. (2015, p. 35) summarised this as follows:

> Complexity emphasizes and incorporates the interconnected, interpenetrating, diverse and sometimes diffuse qualities of most natural and social systems… the nature of things as systemic, complex and affected by particularity of the situations we are in and by the particularity of history.

Complexity theory explores the interplay between current patterns of relationships and the effect of events or variations at particular times and places. Boulton et al. (2015, p. 31) claimed that:

> current patterns form the context in which events may or may not gain impact and so may or may not destabilise them. Thus the future unfolds through the patterns that have been established in the past interacting with current events and variations. The future state of the system is, in this way, path-dependent.

Relating complexity to health and healthcare, Castellani et al. (2015, p. 4) nine requirements of healthcare to perform as a Complex Adaptive System (CAS):

1. A context and composition that is interdependent and causally complex (with circular causality, feedback loops, and concurrent events taking place at multiple levels).
2. The existence of complex, case-based configurations that self-organize and emerge out of the compositional, contextual, and health outcomes factors.
3. The operation of nodes within a network of communities and social forces that recognize the socio-spatial position of places relative to each other and to macroscopic social forces.
4. The presence of dynamic and evolving entities along various socio-spatial trajectories and around different attracting clusters.
5. Impacts that are dynamic and nonlinear.
6. Relationships that are constituted from a mix of historical (institutional memory) and phenomenological (personal, subjective interpretive frames for understanding and participating in a community) factors.
7. Boundaries that are fuzzy, and spatially and sociologically open-ended such that communities are nodes within larger flows of people, places, and things.
8. The ability to negotiate conflicting power struggles among major players and key subsystems (such as community leaders and healthcare systems).
9. An agent-based system comprised of a number of interacting agents that are both mobile and evolving.

The previous chapter explored the role of changes in cognition that can assist implementation of a holistic ecosystem of health and healthcare. This chapter explores the contribution of action to build relationships for collaboration.

9.2 A New Action Paradigm for Health and Healthcare

The World Health Organization has identified that the future of healthcare requires a combination of people, technology (information and medical), and processes (financing, leadership, and governance) (WHO 2007). Cunningham et al. (2012) explained that central to successful action toward this future is recognition of the importance of people and groups of people perceived as actors "with some pattern of interactions or 'ties' between them" (Cunningham et al. 2012, p. 239). This chapter explores a new paradigm of action based in four methods: distributive engagment, networking, participation action (research) and reflexive practice.

The first method of action discussed is that of distributive engagement that aims to build relationships between different expert practitioners and with decision makers.

9.2.1 *Distributive Engagement*

Distributive engagement has been used to underpin a strengths-based approach to identify innovations for future change to address global health challenges. A strengths-based approach replaces the more traditional "deficit" approach that focuses on the need for individuals to fix problems: "professionals, as experts…. observe their subjects and identify their deficits so as to then intervene, address the deficit and solve the problem" (Harvey 2014, p. 732). In contrast, a strengths-based approach is based in the tenet that:

> every individual, every group and every organization has strengths…. Identifying these assets and using them as a starting point for research or practice enables researchers to frame their work within a positive paradigm and build upon these strength. (Harvey 2014, p. 732)

A 'mission-oriented' approach is an example of a strengths-based approach used to address the complexity of global economic challenges (e.g. the global pandemic) (Mazzucato 2020). It does this by interlinking levels of engagement that seek to "catalyze investment and innovation in many different sectors and inspire new collaborations at the project level (Mazzucator 2020, p. 112). First, national (or international) authorities identify a Mission (or Grand Challenge) (Mazzucato 2020, p. 112). Second, a range of experts from many relevant sectors and disciplines are consulted and formed into collaborative teams to undertake research to identify potential innovations to address the Grand Challenge and Mission. Third, agreed proposals for innovations are communicated back to the authorities for final decision (Mazzucato 2018). Five criteria are used to identify the Mission and agree on innovations to be trialled in team projects. Innovations need to be: (i) bold and inspirational with wide societal relevance; (ii) have clear direction with targeted, measurable, and time boundaries; (iii) be ambitious but relevant; iv) engage actors from across disciplines and sectors; and v) have the potential for multiple bottom-up solutions. Through this process of distributive engagement of many experts and decision makers, experimentation and conversations between fundamental and empirical research are fostered.

Two documented examples of the implementation of a distributive mission-oriented approach applied to health and healthcare are the Grand Challenges of "Citizen health and wellbeing" (EU European Commission, EEUC) and "An ageing society" (UK). In the European example, the specific Mission arising from the Grand Challenge was "to decrease the burden of dementia" (Mazzucato 2018). In the UK example, a specific Mission was "to enhance the capabilities and quality of life across the course of our increasingly longer lives" (Mazzucato 2020, p. 120). In both cases, the distributive engagement consisted of engagement of top-down (government decision-makers); middle-out (cross-discipline and cross-sector experts in single-issue research-project teams) and bottom-up (communication of innovative ideas from the research teams back to the decision makers). In the EEUC case, 5 single-issue research project teams were established, each consisting of experts from 9 sectors. In the UK case, 15 single-issue research project teams were established, each consisting of experts from 11 sectors (Mazzucato 2020). The research teams included doctors, social workers, families, designers, teachers, programmers, laboratory workers, pharmaceutical, service and consumer-goods professionals, patients, and those skilled in design and behavioral matters. The issues explored included questions of how to (i) decrease the burden of dementia through a range of self-diagnostic techniques and physical and intellectual support for patients to encourage independence and social standards for caregiving and (ii) enhance capabilities and quality of life through addressing a range of social and economic barriers to mobility and improving diet. This open-ended, distributive, multi-level approach builds relationships between experts and between experts and decision-makers.

However, is silent on the detail of how collaboration between experts is achieved. This leads us to consider a second method of action, of first identifying these experts as nodes and then establishing the means to network them.

9.2.2 *Networking*

The action of networking (often termed, social networking) evolved from innovation theory to explain the spread of new ideas and practices within social systems (Andrews et al. 2013; Callon and Ferrary 2006; Latour 2005; Rogers 2003). Battle-Fisher (2015) described social networks as a "set of relations between objects which could be people, organizations, nations" (p. 3). Kadushin (2012) identified the key assumptions of social network theory as follows:

1. The importance of the aggregate influence of the group.
2. The level of the network at which analysis occurs.
3. Patterns of relationships that exist across the whole network.
4. Relationships that link social networks.

Cunningham et al. (2012, p. 247) claimed that social networks in healthcare provides the opportunity to identify and exploit new knowledge:

> positively functioning networks are likely to contribute more broadly to an effective organisational culture and climate. In this respect, networks can represent not just the social glue of professional interaction but the sociological building blocks of effective organisation.

Social networks have been identified as the source of ideas that flow through social learning. Pentland (2014) explained this as a process in which new ideas take root and change behavior if it is determined that new behavior is likely to be useful. This creates a level of trust and there is some consistency between new ideas and previously learned behaviors.

Social network analysis (SNA) grew from the need to understand the details of what goes on between network nodes. It was initially employed as a "means of mapping and exposing the hidden channels of communication and information flow, collaboration and disconnects between people in strategically important groups within an organisation" (Chambers et al. 2012, p. 1). SNA focuses on identifying relationships that underpin communication, learning, knowledge transfer, and improved decision-making. It works by identifying which nodes to include and then specifying boundaries that include only those nodes (Battle-Fisher 2015). It also enables boundary specifications to be based on positions, events, relations, or reputations (Battle-Fisher 2015).

SNA has been used in healthcare to identify health-professional networks and the structure and sustainability of collaborations and partnerships. It has led to progressive understanding of what networks are, how they are structured, how they operate, and how they develop. However, it is claimed that the effectiveness of networks in sustaining the quality of care and patient safety overtime is uncertain (Cunningham et al. 2012, p. 240). Many healthcare networks have been found to depend on key players, often in management or leadership roles, "who act as connectors to transmit information, bridge disparate groups, liaise across parts of networks and enable social and professional interaction" (Cunningham et al. 2012, p. 247). This focus on key players in SNA has been criticized for its potential vulnerability "if.. [key players]… are relied on excessively and then leave, change roles or become marginalised" (Cunningham et al. 2012, p. 247). This can lead to continuation of embedded hierarchies and network fragmentation (Tasselli 2015). Such criticisms are reduced by actor network theory (ANT).

ANT extends beyond single-player relationships to "locate humans together with material and technical objects inside a complex web of associations" (Bilodeau and Potvin 2016, p. 175). ANT is regarded as suitable for research into health and healthcare given the complexity of population health interventions that often involve partnership and intersectional action (Bilodeau et al. 2011; Potvin and Clavier 2013). ANT provides three advantages for research into health and healthcare:

1. It includes not just actors but the connections between them in an approach that "encompasses and scrutinises the large network of connections supporting or restraining action.... [It] is not the actors per se that comprise the focal point of ANT but rather the connections between them through which they act" (Bilodeau and Potvin 2016, p. 175).
2. It places emphasis on the context in which networks between actors occur; "instead of context being conceived of as a backdrop for networks, intervention contextualization is understood as being the by-product of networks" (Bilodeau and Potvin 2016, p. 175), This contextualization involves:

> identifying the various relevant components in a situation (social actors and their roles, physical objects in the form of material and financial resources, and symbolic objects in the form of scientific or experiential knowledge, values, norms and rules), analysing their attributes, strategic positions and power relationships, points of convergence and divergence with regard to the situation in question, and what is at stake for them, and distinguishing areas of stronger and denser connections

3. It offers an analytical framework through which the effects of intervention can be captured and reconstructed to identify the various connections that allow interventions to change contexts and have impact. This is achieved by being able to illustrate "how effects are produced by connecting various entities (social actors, ideas, facts, resources) that act collectively in a network, and then document the chain of events that produces new connections leading to observed effects" (Bilodeau and Potvin 2016, p. 175). ANT assumes that relationships among and between actors (both human and nonhuman) in an emerging network are mostly unpredictable and affect social environments in ways that are often unexpected.

However, while SNA and ANT emphasise the importance of communicating through networks, they are silent on the actions used to connect the various entities. A third method of action designed to encourage relationships is that of Participatory Action Research.

9.2.3 Participatory Action (Research)

It is argued that designing and managing a process of change within a complexity-framed requires a stepped approach. Boulton et al. (2015) stated that, first, there is need for research into what has shaped the context and what are the strengths of current institutions, patterns, and features, including culture, attitudes, and behaviors. Second, through a process of reflection and interconnection, consideration is given to goals and intentions with broad stakeholder groups. Third, planning and piloting of a project needs to be undertaken that is inclusive of progress reviews that are built in on a regular basis and changed where required. This stepped approach accords with the process of participatory action research (PAR). PAR lends itself to flexible, adaptive, and ongoing emergence of change through spiral steps of planning, action and fact finding, observation, and reflection (Plan, Act, Observe, and

Reflect). It is thus both a philosophy and a methodology of action in which research involves the people engaged in action. Reason and Bradbury (2008) describe PAR as a process that engages practitioners, those affected by services, and researchers in simultaneous action and research (observation and reflection on action). Hughes (2008, p. 390) identifies a PAR process as one of:

> collaboration and participation of co-researchers with different perspectives and ways of understanding, as well as iterative cycles of action and research, provid[ing] a robust model to increase our understanding of complex situations, while designing and monitoring interventions.

As PAR emphasizes cooperative inquiry, it is referred to as being done *with* people, rather than *on* people. It aligns action and research in a more flexible and adaptable manner and thus is relevant and beneficial to the communities directly involved. It is employed in empirical projects as part of an interactive inquiry process that balances problem-solving actions, implemented in a collaborative context, with data-driven collaborative analysis, to seek understanding of underlying causes. This enables predictions about personal and organizational change. Given the need to make sense of emerging patterns, critical reflection provides the opportunity to identify lessons learned as they are actioned and to adjust, adapt, and respond to shifting demands through multiple cycles.

Research in healthcare has traditionally focused on evidenced-based practice (EBP) that relies on using the best available evidence at the time, applying clinical expertise and incorporating consumer-focused healthcare (Sackett et al. 1996). PAR has been applied to EBP to add depth by engaging public and community knowledge and understanding (Viswanathan et al. 2004). PAR has been used, for example, to underpin health promotion (Green et al. 1995) and in hospitals (Waterman et al. 2001). A systematic review of 59 PAR studies by Waterman et al. (2001) found that PAR had been useful in developing innovations, improving health and healthcare, developing knowledge and understanding in practitioners, and involving users and staff. This experience has led to PAR in health and healthcare being identified as: (see Hughes 2008 and Waterman et al. 2001)

1. Generating outcomes that promote generation and development of creative ideas and implementation of changes in practice.
2. Empowering and supporting participants to solve practical, concrete, or material problems and to evaluate change.
3. Contributing to understanding, knowledge, or theory, enabling ongoing feedback through its cyclical process, and educating participants.
4. Acknowledging the complexity of contexts and problems in complex adaptive systems.
5. Providing ethical safeguards as it includes collaboration and participation, both of which are valuable ethical requirement of healthcare practice and research.
6. Including key stakeholders (such as clients, patients, and community members) who are often excluded from decision-making about research.
7. Involving global participants.

8. Supplementing EBP, particularly when clinical decisions require multi-professional teams working on complex problems, new situations, or whole systems, to consider different contexts and purpose.
9. Providing multiple perspectives.
10. Repeating observations and collecting the systematic feedback required to identify emergent patterns that are part of the recognition of health and healthcare as a complex adaptive system and building feedback loops into ongoing research and action.

Norbye (2016) provided a detailed example that highlights the collaborative potential of PAR in a community health services project. The project engaged students from four health-professional programs—nursing, physiotherapy, occupational therapy, and healthcare services—who were formed into interprofessional teams during a 2-week clinical placement. The aims of the project were to explore how students performed interprofessional cooperation in clinical practice and what impact this had on municipal health services. To secure leadership commitment at all levels, the project was designed through collaboration between stakeholders at the university and in healthcare services. Nine different interprofessional groups were established, with a student volunteer from each professional programs. Students negotiated how they would work as a team and suggested different coordination initiatives and how they would learn from each other. Decisions regarding how to work were discussed and agreed upon each workday, with student teams negotiating alternative treatment and care plans with patients and deciding which initiative to implement. Positive feedback from the students engaged in the project included the following:

1. The creation of a positive atmosphere that provided a platform for further work and initiated teamwork.
2. The replacement of stereotypical descriptions of other health professions by deeper understanding of each other's professions.
3. Increased understanding, learning, and willingness to take responsibility for the sharing of knowledge and opinions.
4. Greater patient insight.

The student experience was assessed as contributing to "creating an innovative practice in rural healthcare services … [that] challenged traditional professional ways of thinking and working" (Norbye 2016, p. 8), with the potential to contribute to changes in healthcare services. However, there were doubts about the sustainability of the student experience. The final method of action discussed to build relationships is reflexive practice.[1]

[1] See Chap. 4.

9.2.4 *Reflexive Practice: Knowing-in-Action*

A complex world recognizes the reflexive interaction of elements, or ways that allow feedback which is connected by context. Boulton, Allen, and Bowman (2015, p. 35–36) explained this in the following words:

> you do something to me, and that affects what I do to you and to him, in the light of context which emerged in part out of previous actions and decisions about who did what to whom as result of what was done to them!

Reflective practice has long been acknowledged. In the 1980s, Schön (1983, 1987) proposed an 'epistemology of practice' to extend technical problem-solving to acknowledge the broader context of reflective inquiry and practice, with Shein in later claiming (1996, p. 231) that proposals for change need to be:

> anchored and derive from concrete observations of real behaviour … .hang together and make sense of the data we observe … are amenable to some kind of formal and operational definition so that they can be studied further … provide some link to the concerns of practitioners who are solving real organizational problems here and now.

In focusing on the method of reflexive practice as an action to develop relationships, we are seeking to apply this to describe the process of learning through doing. This acknowledges that reflexive pactice is a way of knowing that is based on experience and action, rather than on abstract concepts or theories. A 'reflexive' practitioner is one who is reflecting and acting simultaneously, exploring and discovering through doing. Reflexivity is thus based on reflecting on one's own experiences and trying to make sense of them, while in action. It is a more passive form of learning that relies heavily on introspection and analysis.

Schmutz and Eppich (2017) highlighted the contribution of reflexivity, given its focus on relational behavior that helps discover, make sense of, and perhaps improve existing patterns and order. Boulton, Allen, and Bowman (2015, p. 5) stated that to understand complexity, there is need to focus not simply on knowledge but on methods, ways of knowing, and ways of acting:

> How do we engage *empirically* with a complex, interconnected, co-evolving, emerging world? How do we learn about how things change? How do we attempt to spot change as it happens? How do we test strategies, work out what has happened and what to do next?

Reflexivity is common in healthcare practice but it is often difficult to identify the separation between reflection and action. Schön (1987) argued that what occurs in healthcare is a continual interweaving of (practical) thinking and (thoughtful) doing, which often take place subconsciously, or as a 'meta-reflection'. However, it can also be applied to the dynamics that occur in research teams, particularly those also using PAR in one of the stages of continuous cycles of change (Ghaye and Lillyman 2010, p. 100). To demonstrate this, Borton (1970) developed a framework for reflective practice based on Kolb's (1984) cycles of experiential learning. This framework highlights the use of observation and reflection on experience to try out new approaches based on the theories as they emerge. The addition of active experimentation allows for the integration of thought and action so that neither makes sense without the other. Borton's reflective framework emphasized three reflective questions: (i) What? (description); (ii) So what? (theorize from description); and (iii) Now what? (plan an active intervention based on the theory generated). In summary, reflexive practice can be seen as an action to build relationships though the identification of how knowledge gained from the (often unconscious) thoughts from practice can be communicated back to influence principles and purpose.

9.3 Discussion: Re-Imagining a Holistic Ecology of Action to Build Relationships

To explore how these four methods of action may assist in developing a new ecology of action to build relationships for collaboration in health and healthcare, the author undertook a four-phase reflective practice approach undertaken by the editors. In the first reflection phase, the four methods of action were examined for their genuineness and comprehensiveness in identifying actions required of the three agencies of health and healthcare: Principles and Purposes (P1); People in Place (P2); and Practices and Processes (P3). The findings, summarised in Table 9.1, are discussed below.

9.3.1 Principles and Purposes (P1)

The first agency (P1) present the opportunity to agree on the underpinning principle and purpose of the collaboration. Linking this to the four methods of action to build relationships identifies the opportunity to encourage: distributive engagement of decision-makers to identify a common goal; networking to develop social systems upon which collaboration for new ideas and practices can occur; PAR to engage agencies in concertive action that results in research *with*, rather than *on*, agencies; and reflexive practice to encourage knowing through interconnected feedback.

9.3.2 People in Place (P2)

The second agency (P2) presents the opportunity to engage people from diverse sectors, levels, and disciplines in research teams. Linking this to the four methods of action to build relationship identifies the opportunity to support: networking to encourage the development of interrelationships between people; PAR to engage a range of experts in empirical practice research through cooperative inquiry; reflexive practice to encourage people to link practice to knowledge development.

Table 9.1 The 3P Agencies of Health and Healthcare: mapping the implications of change in actions to build relationships

3P agencies of health and healthcare	Distributive engagement	Networking	Participatory action research	Reflexive practice
P1 **Principles and Purposes** *Collaboration*	Decision-makers identify a goal.	Social systems become a source of collaboration for new ideas and practice.	Action and research occur in concert *with*, rather than *on*, the researched.	Emphasis is placed on knowing based on doing.
P2 **People in Place** *Interrelated*	Cross-sector, cross-discipline, and multilevel representatives are engaged in research teams.	Linked relationships between nodes are identified.	Participation and joint research in teams are established in situ and engaged in empirical cooperative inquiry.	Knowledge is linked to practice.
P3 **Practices and Processes** *Interconnected*	Practices and processes for bi-directional communication and networking are establised.	Communication and information flows between nodes (people, objects, and associations) are encouraged.	Problem-solving for emergence is encouraged through cycles to develop innovations.	Simultaneous thinking and practice occurs.

9.3.3 Practices and Processes (P3)

The third agency (P3) provides the means to focus on practices and processes to encourage bidirectional communication. Linking this to the four methods of action to build relationships identifies the opportunity to encourage; networking of communication flows between nodes (people, objects, and associations); PAR to focus on a strengths-based problem-solving that encourages emergence through cycles of change; reflexive practice to encourage timely identification of knowledge as it is being constructed.

In the second reflection phase, the potential for interconnection between the four methods of action was considered. This resulted in identification of a potential triangulation of methods in which distributive (top-down, middle-out, bottom-up) engagement establishes the basis upon which relationships can be built while. PAR and reflexive practice, are employed to network with other teams and decision makers to create dynamic, bi-directional interconnected flows of information.

In the third reflection phase consideration was given to how these interconnections can be assembled as a holistic ecology of dynamic action to build relationships for collaboration between the 3Ps. This resulted in the assemblage of an ecology of actions to build relationships, termed the *Distributive Action Relational Ecology (DARE)* illustrated in Fig. 9.1. This highlights the following:

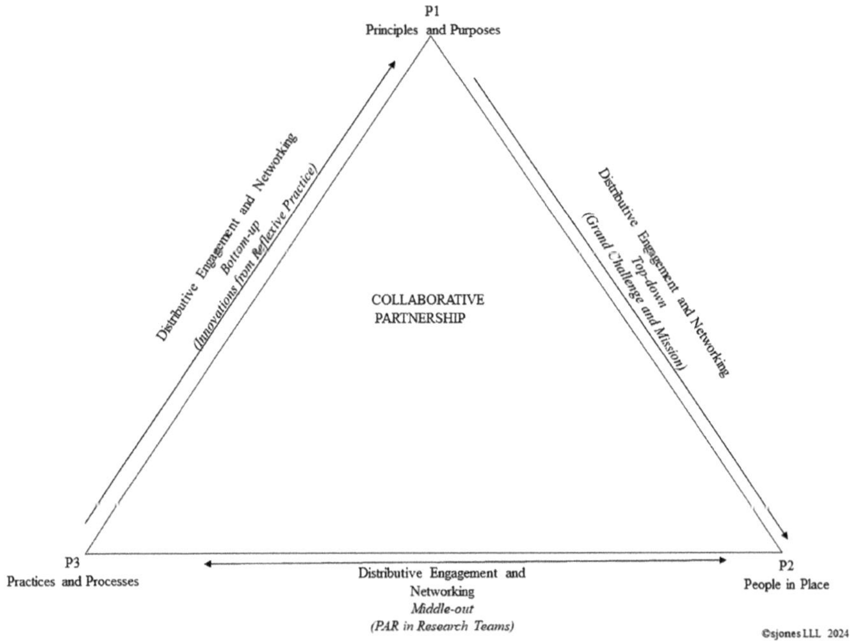

Fig. 9.1 A Distributive Action Relational Ecology (DARE) for Health and Healthcare

1. The importance of *distributive* engagement between each of the agencies with communication and feedback resulting in dynamic interconnections.
2. The value of establishing research teams underpinned by a Participative Action Research processes to encourage knowledge sharing.
3. The contribution of reflexive practice to create the ongoing emergence of knowledge that is networked between the 3P agencies.

Having identified an ecology of actions to build relationships collaboration, the fourth reflection phase aimed to create a resource to assist individuals and groups to design action to encourage understanding of, and commitment to the DARE. This reflection took into account the descriptors of the four methods of action to build relationships for each of the 3Ps. It resulted in the design of a template consisting of 24 reflection prompts (formulated from descriptors of the four methods of action to build relationship) (see Table 9.1) for the 3Ps to consider as appropriate to different contexts. The template is termed the *Self-Enabling Ecology of Reflection on Action* (Template 9.1 *SEER A*).

Template 9.1 Self-Enabling Ecology of Reflection on Action (SEER A)

Use the reflection prompts to identify changes in action to build relationships associated with each of the methods of action…

3P agencies of health and healthcare	Distributive engagement	Social networking	Participatory action research	Reflexive practice
P1 **Principles and purposes** *Collaboration*	*…enable identification of a common principle through top-down, bottom-up and middle-out and*	*…enact understanding of social systems as a source of collaboration for new ideas and practice*	*…enact action and research to occur in concert for collaboration between participants engaged in empirical change*	*…encourage collaboration through knowing based in doing*
P2 **People in place** *Interrelated*	*…encourage cross-sector, cross-discipline and multi-level interrelationship engagement*	*…encourage identification of nodes and the linked relationships between them*	*…encourage participation and research in interrelated teams engaged in empirical cooperative inquiry*	*…enact dynamic change through appreciation of the interrelationships between knowing and doing*
P3 **Practices and processes** *Interconnected*	*…encourage bi-directional inter-communication and networking*	*…encourage interconnections through communication and information flows between nodes (people, objects and associations)*	*…encourage problem-solving for emergence as part of EBP through interconnected cycles to develop innovations*	*…enact simultaneous thinking and practice*

9.4 DARE to CARE

A final reflection phase aimed to identify the interconnecting the four modes of thinking identified in the CARE and the four methods of action identified in the DARE. This resulted in the assemblage of what is termed a DARE to CARE that demonstrates links between cognition and actions to increase collaboration, adaptation and resilience of health and healthcare in complexity. This is illustrated in Fig. 9.2.

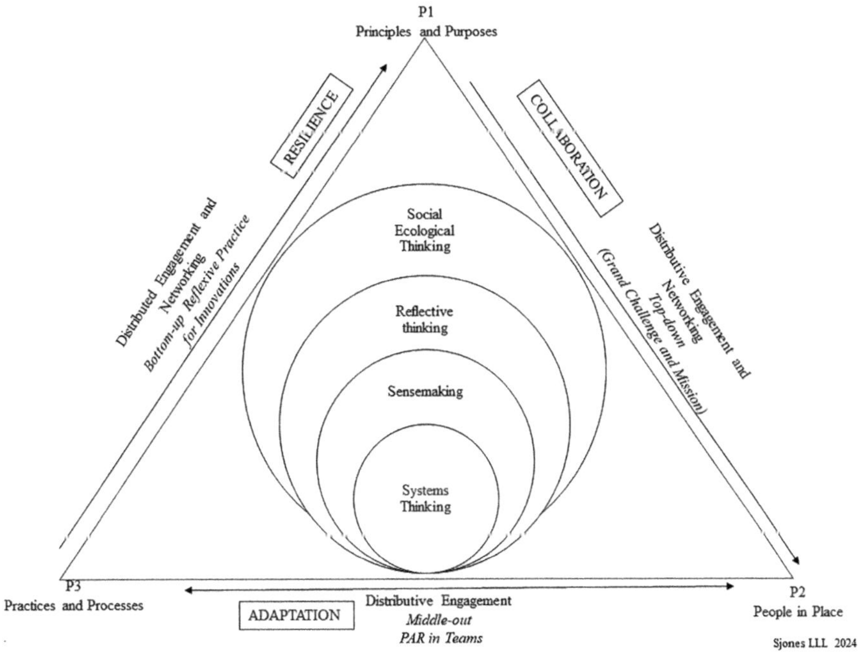

Fig. 9.2 An Action Cognition Ecology (ACE) for Health and Healthcare

9.5 Conclusion

The chapter locates health and healthcare within Complexity science to explore actions to build relationships for collaboration to assist implementation of a holistic ecosystem of health and healthcare. Four methods of action to build relationships were chosen for consideration: distributive engagement, networking, participatory action research and reflexive practice. By employing reflection, the author was able to assemble a dynamic ecology, termed the *Distributive Action Relational Ecology* (*DARE*) for health and healthcare. To assist use of the ecology of action, a resource (termed the *Self-Enabling Ecology on Reflection for Action),* (Template 9.1 *SEER A*) was created. The SEER A can be used by individuals and groups to self identify how to apply the four methods of action to build relationships for collaboration to support a holistic ecosystem of health and healthcare. Finally, the changes in thinking embedded in the change in modes of cognition (CARE) ecology and the methods of action (DARE) identified in this chapter were assembled into one ecology of cognition and action for a holistic ecosystem of health and healthcare.

References

Andrews GJ, Evans J, McAlister S (2013) Creating the right therapy vibe: relational performances in holistic medicine. Soc Sci Med 83:99–109

Battle-Fisher M (2015) Application of systems thinking to health policy & public health ethics, SpringerBriefs in Public Health. Springer. https://doi.org/10.1007/978-3-319-12203-8_1

Bilodeau A, Potvin L (2016) Unpacking complexity in public health interventions with the Actor–Network Theory. Health Promot Int, Debate 33:173–181

Bilodeau A, Galarneau M, Fournier M et al (2011) L'Outil diagnostic de l'action en partenariat: fondements, e'laboration et validation. Can J Public Health 102(4):298–302

Borton T (1970) Reach, touch, teach. McGraw Hill, London

Boulton JG, Allen PM, Bowman C (2015) Embracing complexity: strategic perspectives for an age of turbulence. Oxford University Press

Callon M, Ferrary M (2006) Les re'seaux sociaux a l'aune de la the'orie de l'acteur-re'seau'. Sociologies Pratiques 2(13):37–44

Castellani B, Rjaram R, Buckwalter JG et al (2015) Place and health as complex systems: a case-study and empirical test, SpringerBriefs in Public Health. Springer. https://doi.org/10.1007/978-3-319-09734-3

Chambers D, Wilson P, Thompson C et al (2012) Social networks analysis in healthcare settings: A systematic scoping review. PLoS One 7(8):1-10, e41911

Cunningham FC, Ranmuthugala G, Plumb J et al (2012) Health professional networks as a vector for improving healthcare quality and safety; a systematic review. BMJ Qual Saf 21:239–249

Ghaye T, Lillyman S (2010) Reflection: principles and practices for healthcare professionals. Andrews UK Ltd.

Green LW, George MA, Daniel M et al (1995) Study of participatory research in health promotion: review and recommendations for the development of participatory research in health promotion. Royal Society of Canada, Ottawa, pp 23–34

Harvey M (2014) Strengths-based approach. In: Coghlan D, Brydon-Miller M (eds) The SAGE encyclopaedia of action research, 2nd edn. Sage, Thousand Oaks, pp 732–735

Hughes I (2008) Action research for healthcare, Ch 25. In: Reason P, Bradbury H (eds) Sage handbook of action research, 2nd edn, pp 381–393
Kadushin C (2012) Understanding social networks: theories, concepts, and findings. Oxford University Press
Kolb DA (1984) Experiential learning: experiences on the source of learning and development. Prentice Hall, Hoboken
Latour B (2005) Reassembling the social. An introduction to actor-network-theory. Oxford University Press, New York
Mazzucato M (2018) Mission -oriented research and innovation in the European Union. European Commission, Director General for Research and Innovation, Brussels
Mazzucato M (2020) Mission economy. Penguin Random House, UK
Norbye B (2016) Healthcare students as innovative partners in the development of future healthcare services: an action research approach. Nurse Educ Today 46:4–9
Pentland A (2014) Social physics. Scribe Publications, Brunswick Victoria and Sans Way London
Potvin L, Clavier C (2013) Actor-network theory: the governance of intersectoral initiatives. In: Clavier C, De Leeuw E (eds) Health promotion and the policy process. Oxford University Press, Oxford, pp 82–103
Reason P, Bradbury H (eds) (2008) Sage handbook of action research, 2nd edn SAGE
Rogers EM (2003) Diffusion of innovations. Free Press, New York and London
Sackett DL, Rosenberg WMC, Muir GJ, A. et al (1996) Evidence-based medicine: what it is and what it isn't. Br Med J 312:71–72
Schein E (1996) Culture: the missing concept in organizations studies. Adm Sci Q 41:229–240
Schmutz JB, Eppich WJ (2017) Promoting learning and patient care through shared reflection: a conceptual framework for team reflexivity in health care. Acad Med 92(11):1555–1563
Schön D (1983) The reflective practitioner: how professionals think in action. Basic Books, New York
Schön D (1987) Educating the reflective practitioner. Jossey-Base, San Francisco
Tasselli S (2015) Social networks and interprofessional knowledge transfer: the case of healthcare professionals. Organ Stud 36(7):841–872
Viswanathan M, Ammerman A, Eng E et al (2004) Community based participatory research: assessing the evidence. Evidence Report/Technology Assessment No. 99 (No. AHRQ Publication 04-E022-2). Rockville, MD: Agency for Healthcare Research and Quality
Waterman H, Tillen D, Dickson R et al (2001) Action research: a systematic review and guidance for assessment. Health Technol Assess 5(23):1–166
World Health Organization (WHO) (2007) Everybody's business: strengthening health systems to improve health outcomes: WHO's Framework for Action

Chapter 10
A Holistic Ecosystem of Health and Healthcare: Leading Change

Sandra Jones

Abstract The aim of this chapter is to discuss and reflect on changes in approach to leadership to encourage collaboration that are aligned with the principles of Complexity science for a holistic ecosystem of health and healthcare. It first discusses three theories of leadership: Ecological Leadership, Systems Leadership, and Distributed Leadership. It then analyzes the implications of these three theories for the three agencies of health and healthcare: Principles and Purposes (P1); People in Place (P2); and Practices and Processes (P3). The outcome is the assemblage of an ecology of lead(er) ship, termed the Dynamic Lead(er)ship Ecology of Adaptive Partnerships (LEAP) that is designed to encourage collaboration, adaptation and relationships. Finally, it reflects upon the link between the modes of cognition, methods of action to build relationships, and approach to lead(er)ship, resulting in the assemblage of an ecology of cognition, action and lead(er)ship, termed the Action Cognition Ecology (ACE) of Lead(er)ship for health and healthcare.

10.1 Self-Organizing Systems in Complexity

Adopting a complexity worldview requires working with a wide group of stakeholders who are close to what is happening. It assumes that, given this closeness, the stakeholders are more likely to recognize what is working well and what is not, and what is changing. Such a change in focus raises the question of the role, and nature, of leadership. Boulton, Allen, and Bowman (2015, p. 136) claimed that:

> in general there is need for leaders to *handle ambiguity* and to handle complex information and to be able to synthesise out of that a sense of how to create a way forward—to see a path through the woods emerging out of the trees….part of the role of leadership is to provide tasks and conditions in which people can have enough certainty to 'get on with things'. Whilst at the same time designing processes through which unexpected outcomes and new issues on the horizon may be notices and considered.

S. Jones (✉)
Business and Law College, RMIT University, Melbourne, VIC, Australia

S. Jones, D. Vindigni OAM (eds.), *Health and Healthcare in Complexity*,
https://doi.org/10.1007/978-981-96-0515-6_10

Complexity places emphasis on self-organization that comes from within rather than being imposed from outside or 'top-down.' In this self-organization, leadership is viewed as only one of a gamut of factors alongside "history, context, relationships and existing patterns and processes that together contribute to what form results" (Boulton, Allen and Bowman (2015, p. 45). Leadership comes to be seen as an activity, rather than a role, requiring a new range of competencies. Rather than a focus on individual competencies to make decisions, leadership becomes how to inspire others (look forward); to anticipate (critical junctures), to adapt (deal with dynamism and uncertainty), and to customize (respond to unique contexts). At the same time to encourage greater autonomy. This is explained by Boulton et al. 2015, p. 6) as the need to:

> focus on the initial selection of good professionals, allowing them more autonomy to respond more effectively to the situations they are facing … [rather than]… the considerable efforts put in by managers to direct, measure and control their performance. If the world is complex, then acting congruently with that complexity can be simpler that trying to control a machine that does not exist.

10.2 A New Paradigm of Leadership for Health and Healthcare

The impact of complexity on leadership for health and healthcare has been to challenge the traditional hierarchical approach to encourage broad engagement of a diverse array of experts. Plsek and Wilson (2001 p. 749) stated that:

> effective organisation and delivery of healthcare does not need detailed targets and specifications, nor should it focus primarily on 'controlling the process' or 'overcoming resistance.' Rather, those who seek to change an organisation should harness the natural creativity and organising ability of its staff and stakeholders through such principles as generative relationships, minimum specification, the positive use of attractors for change, and a constructive approach to variation in areas of practice where there is only moderate certainty and agreement

Sturmberg, O'Halloran, and Martin (2010, p. 474) reinforced this with their claim that agents in a Complex Adaptive System:

> self organise around a core driver…are sensitive to initial conditions, and often display non-linear dynamics…. Agents in dynamic networks are constantly acting and reacting in response to other agents…the observed overall behaviour of the system is the result of a huge number of "decision" and "actions" taken every moment by individual agents.

This contrasts with the traditional administrative hierarchy that has characterised healthcare management that has been grounded in the mechanistic (Newtonian influenced) concept of scientific management (Snowden and Boone 2007). O'Reilly and Reed (2010) used the term "leaderism" to describe traditional healthcare leadership that is grounded in individuals (De Brún and McAuliffe 2020; Bolden et al. 2006; Davidson 2010; Dickinson and Ham 2008). While it is claimed that hierarchies can be beneficial in cases where issues need to be clarified, or in emergencies when tasks need to be assigned quickly, it is argued that they have limited value in the complex world of clinical leadership (McKimm 2011). This has led to hierarchies in health and healthcare being criticized for the following:

1. Creating tensions and negatively affecting teamwork and patient care by allowing fear and intimidation to discourage respectful communication (Clapper 2018).
2. Not addressing the "highly complex interrelated relationship-driven characteristics of healthcare organisations" (Hartviksen et al. 2018, p. 2).
3. Producing negative outcomes such as "serious care failures and shortfalls in performance relative to expectations" (Beirne 2017, p. 2).
4. Shaping an organizational culture focused on performance evaluation of individual (leader) behaviors rather than on the design of strategies and qualities to improve health service (West et al. 2015).
5. Fostering a culture of fear and blame (Hartmann et al. 2009) rather than a culture of sustainable improvement in quality, safety, and patient outcomes (Beirne 2017; Kaufman and McCaughan 2013).

In response several, more collaborative approaches to leadership for health and healthcare have been the subject of discussion. The theories of leadership chosen for discussion in this chapter are: Ecological Leadership, Distributed Leadership and Systems Leadership.

10.2.1 Ecological Leadership

Ecological leadership is a form of leadership that changes the focus from individuals to the reciprocal interactions between people. In so doing it flattens hierarchies and emphasizes networks between people, objects, and symbols (biological, psychological, and contextual). This requires leadership to be viewed as a relational activity (Allen et al. 1998) in which leaders are exhorted to:

1. Acknowledge the multiple talents and capacities of people.
2. Enact effective processes and system to engage people.
3. Develop behaviors aimed at using all relevant expertise.
4. Encourage equality.
5. Establish the means to evaluate adaptability and response to long term challenges.
6. Balance tensions between competing values (Wielkiewicz and Stelzner 2005).

Hurst (2012) described Ecological Leadership as requiring leaders to acknowledge a values-based "social 'ecologic' of people" (Hurst 2012, p. 110). This to be achieved through action to "encourage exchange and reciprocity in relationships, re-engage people's senses by encouraging them to story-tell the past…and then connect them together in webs of cause and effect" (Hurst 2012, p. 3).

However, despite discussion of the need to engage more people, advocates of ecological leadership retain the focus on individuals in positions of leadership (Leach et al. 2021, p. 355). Individual leaders are exhorted to be mindful and communicative, to focus on building collaborative relationships that engage synergistically with the environment (Van Vactor 2012), and to take more notice of employee expertise (Hurst 2012). There are few examples of ecological leadership viewed from an activity perspective in which the focus is on the many people (including formally designated leaders) engaged in the work of leadership (Davis and Jones 2014; Jones 2022, 2023).

Ongoing concern about the negative outcomes of a single-leader approaches have led to interest in more collective, often termed "post-heroic," leadership (Fletcher 2004). Collectivist approaches to leadership have been described as leadership in which "roles and responsibilities are shared, distributed or rotated amongst team members" (De Brún et al. 2019, p. 1). Teams have been encouraged to include representatives from the same or different disciplines, professions, or units (Denis et al. 2001; Chreim and MacNaughton 2016). A plethora of theories have emerged under the umbrella of collective leadership, including complexity leadership (Uhl-Bien et al. 2007), relational leadership (Fletcher and Kaufer 2003; Uhl-Bien 2006; Fulop and Mark 2013), shared leadership (Pearce and Conger 2003; Bolden et al. 2015), distributed leadership (Gronn 2000; Bolden 2011; Jones 2020), hybrid leadership (Gronn 2009, 2011), collective leadership (Ospina 2017; Bolden et al. 2008), and systems leadership (Bolden et al. 2019; Ghate et al. 2013; Senge et al. 2015). However, while these theories advocate a collectivist approach to leadership, most retain the focus on individual leaders.

Two exceptions, both of which have been trialed in healthcare, are Distributed Leadership and Systems Leadership. Both these theories view leadership as inclusive of experts and formally designated leaders rather than dependent on a few making decisions at the top that are filtered down (Bigland et al. 2020; Jones 2020).

10.2.2 Distributed Leadership

In Chap. 7 we discussed that during the early 2000s several national governments (UK, Australia and Canada) encouraged the adoption of Distributed Leadership for healthcare. However it was acknowledged that this had limited impact and was not sustained. Over a similar period of time, Higher Education (in the UK and Australia) had a similar experience of Distributed Leadership (see Bolden et al. 2008; Jones et al. 2012, 2014; and Bolden et al. 2015)[1]. However, in the case of higher education, more detailed research was undertaken into the elements that contribute to Distributed Leadership.[2] In the UK, four principle elements were identified:

1. Alignment of top-down, bottom-up, and horizontal leadership, although the challenges of achieving this balance were recognized.

[1] It was also discussed in the USA, but in this case, it retained a single-leader focus.

[2] Higher education is an important source of new graduates to healthcare, often educated by healthcare professionals and undertaking their practice-based education in healthcare.

2. Acknowledgement and encouragement of informal networks and relationships.
3. Action that inspires a sense of common purpose and direction, engenders a sense of trust and openness, encourages communication and dialog, and creates an innovative and supportive culture in which initiative can flourish.
4. Provision of more personalized support through mentoring, coaching, and development opportunities (Bolden et al. 2008).

In Australia, where Distributed Leadership was described as the "engagement of many individuals based on their various expertise, through which collaborative relationships are built" (Jones 2020, p. 379), six tenets of Distributed Leadership were identified:

1. *Engage* a broad range of positional leaders and experts.
2. *Enable* through a context and culture of trust, respect, and collaboration.
3. *Enact* via a holistic approach that includes processes and systems designed to encourage the involvement of people.
4. *Encourage* through support for professional development that includes mentoring and facilitation, finance, recognition, and reward.
5. *Evaluate* outcomes against aims.
6. *Emergence* fostered through ongoing cycles of change as a strengths-based approach built on lessons learned, (Jones et al. 2014).

These tenets have since been tested for their applicability in a range of contexts and cultures, including healthcare.[3]

10.2.3 Systems Leadership

Extending the research into Distributed Leadership in higher education, in the UK research was undertaken into Systems Leadership, particularly in public health. Systems leadership is described as focusing "beyond professional boundaries in order to address cross-cutting 'wicked' problems" (Bigland et al. 2020, p. 2). In adding the focus on integration between the professions this research focuses on *themes*, rather than professional boundaries, each identified by a range of activities:

1. Common commitment to an issue-based (rather than leader-centric) approach.
2. Three phases (themes), termed *assembling a coalition of the willing*, *maintaining momentum*, and *indicators of success*.
3. Sets of activities for each phase that include systems, processes, and behaviors, related to activities such as building trust and reciprocal relations and developing behaviors to work together in uncertainty (Bolden et al. 2019).

[3] For example, see Jones 2020, 2022, 2023; Harvey and Jones 2022, 2021; and Jones and Harvey 2017.

10.3 Discussion: An Ecology of Lead(er)ship for Health and Healthcare

To explore how these three approaches to leadership may assist in developing a new ecology of leadership for health and healthcare, the editors undertook a four-phase reflective practice approach. In the first, reflection phase, the three approaches to leadership were examined for their genuineness and comprehensiveness in identifying changes required of the three agencies of health and healthcare: Principles and Purposes (P1); People in Place (P2) and Practices and Processes (P3). The findings, summarised in Table 10.1, are discussed below:

10.3.1 Principles and Purposes (P1)

The first agency (P1) identifies common acceptance of the need for leadership to be reconceptualized away from an individual position to being seen as engaging many experts, within and across professions, in the activity of leadership. This to be achieved assuming an issue based approach and encouraging informal networks and relationships.

10.3.2 People in Place (P2)

The second agency (P2) acknowledges the importance of encouraging people with a multitude of talents and capacities within, and between, professions and organizations to participate in leadership: Systems Leadership emphasizes the importance of *assembling a coalition of the willing* to ensure that action is undertaken to align personal and professional values, interests, and behaviors; Distributed Leadership captures this under the tenet of *engage* through which experts and decision-makers work together to incorporate top-down, bottom-up, and horizontal (middle-out) views.

Both Systems and Distributed Leadership also acknowledge the importance of developing a supportive context and culture that encourages cooperation through actions designed to achieve a balance between competing forces, tensions, actions, and contexts. In adopting an issue-based, cross discipline focus, Systems Leadership identifies a detailed list of action needed that include: appointment of a systems coordinator to facilitate a process that builds and maintains relationships through a culture of inclusivity, diversity, reciprocal trust, and respect and conflict resolution through constructive discussion, perseverance, and intellectual challenge. Distributed leadership captures this under the tenet of *enable*, through which a context and culture of trust, respect, and commitment to change is encouraged by common purpose and direction.

10.3.3 Practices and Processes (P3)

The third agency (P3) acknowledges the significance of joint commitment to develop practices, systems, and processes that support the engagement of people. This includes the following:

(i) Employment of systems to encourage equality between employees; Systems Leadership describes this under the theme of *maintaining the momentum* in which actions are taken to balance autocracy and democracy appropriate to responding to uncertainty, conflict, and paradox as well as taking advantage of serendipity to build resilience. Distributed Leadership captures this under the tenet of *enact*, through which systems are designed to encourage involvement, communication, and dialog for innovation.

(ii) Design of processes to ensure that leaders develop skills of adaptability to different contexts: Systems Leadership describes actions needed to encourage an open mindset to build trust and safety and encourage curiosity by focusing on understanding through listening. Distributed Leadership captures this under the tenet of *encourage* through which awareness is raised through communication, professional development, mentoring, and coaching.

(iii) Development of new measures to assess outcomes of engagement. Systems Leadership employs the phrase *indicators of success* to emphasize the need to broaden assessment to include measures of enjoyment and alignment of values, and impact. This includes stories, recognition through awards, and the ongoing attraction of funding. Distributed Leadership captures this under the tenet of *evaluate* outcomes against aims and the tenet of *emergence* through cycles of chance through which "the final state is radically and qualitatively different from the starting state" (Boulton et al. 2015, p. 45).

In the second reflection phase, the potential to align the themes and actions identified for Systems Leadership to encourage an issue-based cross professions approach and the tenets of Distributed Leadership was explored. The outcome was identification of an alignment between the two, albeit with the emphasis changing from within a single profession or organization, to cross discipline and professional collaborative partnerships underpinned by an issue-based focus. With this additional focus (proviso) the 6E tenets of Distributed Leadership were adapted to correlate with the 'themes' of Systems Leadership. This led to the assemblage of a dynamic ecology, termed the *Lead(er)ship Ecology of Adaptive Partnerships (LEAP)* of health and healthcare as illustrated in Fig. 10.1. This highlights the following:

1. The importance of *enabling* leadership that *engages* people to '*assemble a coalition of the willing*' from many contexts, cultures, professions and disciplines. Adopting an issue-based approach encourages a sense of common purpose and direction to build and maintain respectful relationships built on trust, diversity, and inclusiveness.
2. The value of *encouraging* engagement through *enacting* supportive systems and processes that encourage active participation and '*maintain the momentum*' by

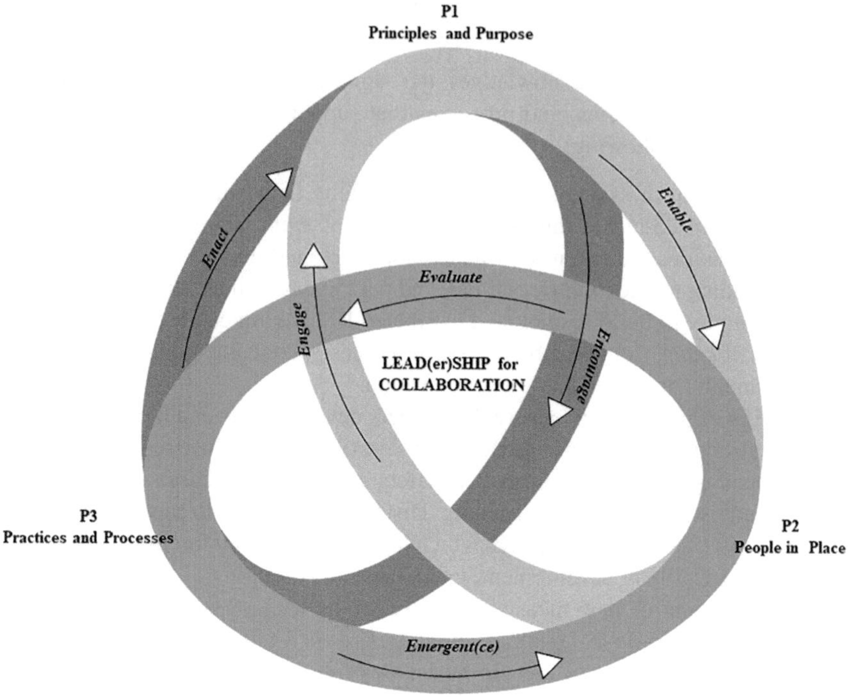

Fig. 10.1 A Lead(er)ship Ecology of Adaptive Partnerships (LEAP) for Health and Healthcare

developing systems able to build support to live with paradox, create conditions for serendipity and build resistence.

3. The significance of designing new measures as '*indicators of success*' to *evaluate* collaboration based in measures of enjoyment and alignment of values that recognise and reward work. The outcome being to encourage *emergence* through cycles of change that may attract ongoing support.

Having identified an ecology of lead(er)ship, a third reflection phase was undertaken with the aim of creating a resource to assist individuals and groups to identify opportunities to engage many experts in the work of lead(er)ship appropriate to specific contexts and cultures. The reflection took into account the descriptors of each of the three approaches to leadership. This resulted in the design of a resource with 21 reflection prompts (formulated from the descriptors of the three approaches to leadership), (see Table 10.1) for the 3Ps, termed the *Self-Enabling Ecology of Reflection* on Lead(er)ship (Template 10.1 *SEER L*).

Table 10.1 The 3P Agencies of Health and Healthcare: mapping the implications of a change in lead(er)ship

3P agencies of health and healthcare	Ecology of Leadership	Systems Leadership	Distributed Leadership
P1 Principles and Purposes	Establish a relational role of leaders in leadership	Establish an issue-based rather than leader-centric focus	Acknowledge activity that encourages informal networks and relationships
P2 People in Place	Use the multitude of talent and capacities within the organization	***Assemble a coalition of the willing*** • Align personal and professional values • Attract people with interest, time, and funding • Encourage behaviors of perseverance and intellectual challenge	***Engage*** Experts and decision-makers aligned with a *top-down*, *bottom-up*, and *horizontal processes*
	Emphasize cooperation to balance competing forces, tensions, actions, and context	• Build and maintain relationships • Build a culture of inclusivity and diversity, value, and respect • Resolve conflict by constructive discussion	***Enable*** Context and culture of trust and respect and commitment to change *Inspired by a sense of common purpose and direction and sense of trust and openness*
P3 Practices and Processes (i) Systems	Encourage equality	***Maintain momentum*** • Institute a systems coordinator • Develop systems that can live with paradoxes to balance autocracy and democracy • Create conditions for serendipity • Build resilience through support	***Enact*** Processes and systems designed to implement change
(ii) Processes	Evaluate for adaptability to changing contexts	• Prepare leaders to work together to build trust and safety • Encourage curiosity, an open mindset, and capacity to live with uncertainty	***Encourage*** Raise awareness and scaffold understanding through personalized support, mentoring, coaching, and development
(iii) Assessments	Foster leadership that champions emergence	***Indicators of success*** • Develop measures of enjoyment and alignment of values that recognize and reward work • Attract ongoing cumulative funding	***Evaluate*** Outcomes against aims ***Emergence*** Through cycles of change

© SJones LLL, 2024

Template 10.1 Self-Enabling Ecology of Reflection on Lead(er)ship (SEER L)

Use the reflection prompts to identify changes to acknowledge lead(er)ship as an activity to encourage

3P agencies of health and healthcare	*…ENABLE…*	*…ENGAGE…*	*…ENACT…*	*…ENCOURAGE…*	*…EVALUATE…*	*…FOSTER EMERGENCE…*
P1 Principles and purposes	*…the work of lead(er)ship*	*…in relationships based on values of inclusivity and diversity*	*…collaboration as part of a collective*	*…understanding of lead(er)ship*	*…by identifying means to demonstrate outcomes against aims*	
P2 People in place	*…alignment of personal and professional values*	*…people with expertise, interest, time and funding*	*…a coalition of the willing with perseverance and commitment to intellectual growth*	*…awareness and understanding of collaboration …curiosity, an open mindset and communication for understanding*	*…by adding measures of enjoyment and alignment of values*	*…by creating conditions for serendipity*
P3 Practices and processes (i) Systems	*…the balancing of autocracy and democracy*	*…diverse individuals by actions to…*	*…the design of systems for conflict resolution to prepare participants to work together*	*…two-way communication and understanding*	*…by identifying impact through stories*	*…by implementing cycles of change*
(ii) Processes	*…living with uncertainty*	*…in processes to maintain momentum over time*	*…collaboration in relationships*	*…structural support to build resilience*	*…by recognising and rewarding contribution*	*…by attracting ongoing cumulative funding*

10.4 Integrating Cognition, Action, and Lead(er)ship: The ACE of DARE to CARE

Having assembled three ecologies to identify change in modes of cognition, methods of action, and forms of lead(er)ship, a final reflection phase was undertaken to identify interconnections between the four modes of thinking, the four methods of action and the proposed approach to lead(er)ship. This resulted in the identification of a complementary multilayered holistic ecology, termed the Action Cognition Ecology (ACE) of Lead(er)ship for collaboration in health and healthcare (Fig. 10.2), that acknowledges the following:

1. The importance of developing trust and respect for collaboration through cognitive change that places emphasis on *enabling* commitment to a common principle and purpose.
2. The goal of collaboration achieved through the distributive engagement of a diversity of participants with different forms of expertise.
3. The value of adopting a mix of cognitive, action-based relational and leadership changes that *enact* collaboration.
4. The significance of participation and networking in teams and groups employing modes of thinking that *encourage* collaboration.
5. The importance of identifying new means to *evaluate* adaptation for collaboration through new forms of thinking and sensemaking.
6. The usefulness of emphasizing ongoing emergence from the mix of cognitive change and participative action and reflection.

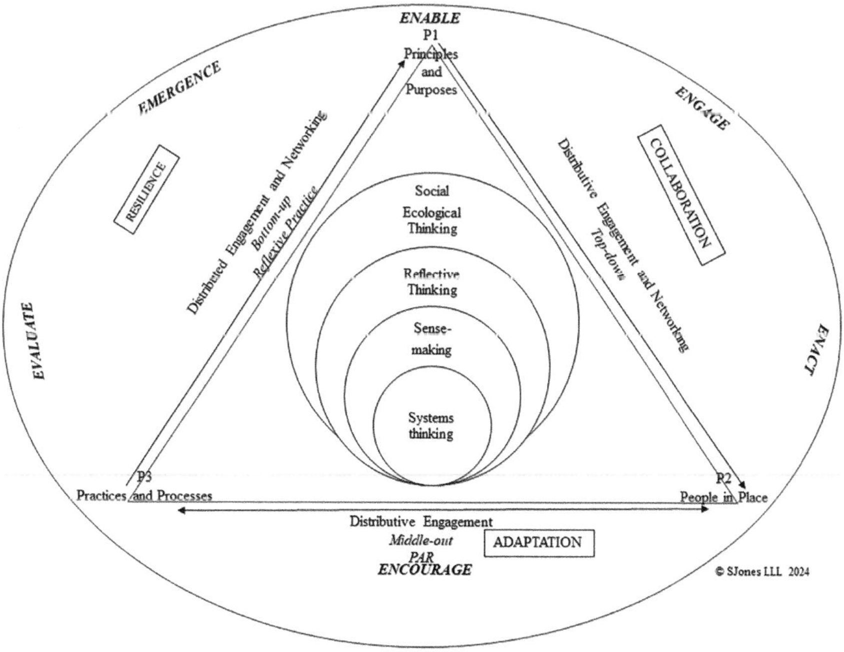

Fig. 10.2 An Action Cognition Ecology of Lead(er)ship (ACEL) for Health and Healthcare

10.5 Conclusion

This chapter locates leadership for health and healthcare within Complexity science to explore actions to encourage leadership that engage many (intra and cross-professional) experts to assist implementation of collaboration within a holistic ecology of health and healthcare. Three approaches to leadership were chosen for detailed exploration: Ecological Leadership; Systems Leadership and Distributed Leadership. By employing a reflective approach, a dynamic ecology of lead(er)ship, termed the *Lead(er)ship Ecology of Adaptive Partnerships (LEAP),* was assembled. To assist the translation of the new approach to leadership, a resource in the form of a *Self-Enabling Ecology of Reflection on Lead(er)ship (SEER L)* was designed. Finally, the potential to interconnect the three ecologies of cognition, action and lead(er)ship resulted in the assemblage of a multilayered Action, Cognition Ecology (ACE) of Lead(er)ship for collaboration in health and healthcare.

References

Allen K, Stelzner SP, Wielkiewicz RM (1998) The ecology of leadership: adapting to the challenges of a changing world. J Leadersh Stud 5(2):62–81

Beirne M (2017) The reforming appeal of distributed leadership. British Journal of Healthcare Management 19(1):72. https://doi.org/10.1186/s12913-019-3883-x

Bigland C, Evans D, Bolden R (2020) Systems leadership in practice: thematic insights from three public health case studies. BMC Public Health 20:1735. https://doi.org/10.1186/s12889-020-09641-1

Bolden R (2011) Distributed leadership in organizations: a review of theory and research. Int J Manag Rev 13(3):251–269. https://doi.org/10.1111/ijmr.2011.13.issue-3

Bolden R, Wood M, Gosling J (2006) Is the NHS leadership qualities framework missing the wood from the trees? In: Casebeer AL, Harrison A, Mark AL (eds) Innovations in health care: a reality check. Palgrave Macmillan, Basingstoke, Hampshire, pp 17–29

Bolden R, Petrov G, Gosling J (2008) Developing collective leadership in higher education, Final report. Research and Development Series. Leadership Foundation for Higher Education, London

Bolden R, Jones S, Davis H et al (2015) Developing and sustaining shared leadership. Stimulus paper. Leadership Foundation for Higher Education & L. H. Martin Institute. https://www.advance-he.ac.uk/knowledge-hub/developing-and-sustaining-shared-leadership-higher-education

Bolden R, Evans D, Jarvis C et al (2019) Developing system leadership in public health. A scoping report. UWE Bristol, Bristol

Boulton JG, Allen PM, Bowman C (2015) Embracing complexity: strategic perspectives for an Age of Turbulence. Oxford University Press

Chreim S, MacNaughton K (2016) Distributed leadership in health care teams: constellation role distribution and leadership practices. Health Care Manag Rev 41(3):200–212

Clapper TC (2018) TeamSTEPPS® is an effective tool to level the hierarchy in healthcare communication by empowering all stakeholders. J Communication in Healthcare. 11(4):241–244

Davidson SJ (2010) Complex responsive processes: a new lens for leadership in twenty-first-century health care. Nursing Forum 45(2):108–117. Malden, USA: Blackwell Publishing Inc

Davis H, Jones S (2014) The work of leadership in higher education management. J High Educ Policy Manag 36(4):367–370. http://www.tandonline.com/doi/full/10.1080/1360080X.2014.916469

De Brún A, McAuliffe E (2020) Identifying the context, mechanisms and outcomes underlying collective leadership in teams: building a realist programme theory. BMC Health Serv Res 20:1–13. https://doi.org/10.1186/s12913-020-05129-1

De Brún A, O'Donovan R, McAuliffe E (2019) Interventions to develop collectivistic leadership in healthcare settings: a systematic review. BMC Health Serv Res 19:1–22

Denis JL, Lamothe L, Langley A (2001) The dynamics of collective leadership and strategic change in pluralistic organizations. Acad Manag J 44(4):809–837

Dickinson H, Ham C (2008) Engaging doctors in leadership: review of the literature. University of Birmingham, Academy of Medical Royal Colleges, NHS Institute for Innovation Improvement, Birmingham UK

Fletcher JK (2004) The paradox of postheroic leadership: an essay on gender, power and transformational change. Leadership Quarterly 15(5):647–661

Fletcher JK, Kaufer K (2003) Shared leadership: paradox and possibilities. In: Pearce C, Conger J (eds) Shared leadership: reframing the hows and whys of leadership. Sage Publications, Thousand Oaks, CA, pp 21–47

Fulop L, Mark A (2013) Relational leadership, decision-making and the messiness of context in healthcare. Leadership 9(2):254–277

Ghate D, Lewis J, Welbourn D (2013) Systems leadership: exceptional leadership for exceptional times-synthesis report. Virtual Staff College, Nottingham

Gronn P (2000) Distributed properties. Educ Manag Adm Leadersh 28(3):317–338

Gronn P (2009) Leadership configurations. Leadership 5(3):381–394

Gronn P (2011) Hybrid configurations of leadership. The Sage handbook of leadership: 437–454.

Hartmann CW, Meterko M, Rosen AK et al (2009) Relationship of hospital organizational culture to patient safety climate in the veterans health administration. Med Care Res Rev 66(3):320–338

Hartviksen T, Sjolie B, Aspfors J, Uhrenfeldt L (2018) Healthcare middle managers experiences developing leadership capacity and capability in a public funded learning network. BMC Health Sci Res 18:433. https://doi.org/10.1186/s12913-018-3259-7

Harvey M. Jones S (2021) Enabling leadership capacity for higher education scholarship in learning and teaching (SOTL) through action research. Educational Action Research 29(2):173–190

Harvey M, Jones S (2022) Challenge Accepted: Women Claiming Leadership in Higher Education Learning and Teaching. Journal of University Teaching and Learning Practice. 19(1):68–89

Hurst D (2012) The new ecology of leadership: business mastery in a chaotic world. Columbia University Press, New York

Jones S, Harvey M (2017) A distributed leadership change process model for higher education. Journal of Higher Education Policy and Management 39(2):126–139.

Jones S (2020) Distributed leadership. In David M.E, Amey M.J (eds) SAGE encyclopedia of higher education: 378–381, Thousand Oaks: SAGE Publications

Jones S (2022) Valuing collaboration in leadership in learning and teaching, Ch 10. In: Rao N, Hosein A, Kinchin I (eds) Narratives of academics' personal journey in contested spaces: leadership identity in learning and teaching in higher education, Part III Engaging values, resilience and serendipity in leadership. Bloomsbury Publishing, pp 163–178

Jones S (2023) An ecological view of distributed leadership for higher education. In: International perspectives on leadership in higher education, vol 15. Emerald Publishing Limited, pp 255–269. https://doi.org/10.1108/S1479-362820220000015014. ISSN: 1479-3628

Jones S, Harvey M, Lefoe G et al (2012) Lessons learnt: identifying synergies in distributed leadership projects Final report. Office for Learning and Teaching. https://ltr.edu.au/resources/LE9_1222_Jones_Report_2012.pdf

Jones S, Hadgraft R, Harvey M, Lefoe G et al (2014) Evidence-based benchmarking framework for a distributed leadership approach to capacity building in learning and teaching Final report. OLT. https://ltr.edu.au/resources/LE11_2000_Jones_Report_2014_0.pdf

Kaufman G, McCaughan D (2013) The effect of organisational culture on patient safety. Nurs Stand 27(43):50

Leach L, Hastings B, Schwarz G et al (2021) Distributed leadership in healthcare: leadership dyads and the promise of improved hospital outcome. Leadersh Health Serv 34(4):353–374

McKimm J (2011) Leading for collaboration and partnership working. In: Swanwick T, McKimm J (eds) ABC of clinical leadership. Wiley Blackwell, Chichester, pp 44–49

O'Reilly D, Reed M (2010) 'Leaderism': an evolution of managerialism in UK public sector reforms. Public Adm 88(4):960–978

Ospina S (2017) Collective leadership and context in public administration: bridging public leadership research and leadership studies. Public Adm Rev 77(2):275–287

Pearce CL, Conger JA (2003) Shared leadership: Reframing the hows and whys of leadership. SAGE Publications, Inc, pp 1–18

Plsek PE, Wilson T (2001) Complexity, leadership, and management in healthcare organisations. BMJ 323(7315):746–749

Senge P, Hamilton H, Kania J (2015) The dawn of systems leadership. Stanf Soc Innov Rev 13(1):26–33

Snowden DJ, Boone ME (2007) A leader's framework for decision making. Harv Bus Rev 85(11):68–76

Sturmberg JP, O'Halloran DM, Martin CM (2010) People at the centre of complex adaptive health systems reform. MJA 193(8):474–478

Uhl-Bien M (2006) Relational leadership theory: exploring the social processes of leadership and organizing. Leadersh Q 17(6):654–676

Uhl-Bien M, Marion R, McKelvey B (2007) Complexity leadership theory: shifting leadership from the industrial era to the knowledge. Leadersh Q 18(4):293–318

Van Vactor J (2012) Collaborative leadership model in the management of health care. J Bus Res 65:555–561

West M, Armit K, Loewenthal L et al (2015) Leadership and leadership development in health care: the evidence base. The Kings Fund, London

Wielkiewicz RM, Stelzner SP (2005) An ecological perspective on leadership theory, research and practice. Rev Gen Psychol 9(4):326–341

Chapter 11
Learning from the Wisdoms of Indigenous Elders

Dein Vindigni OAM, Uncle Paul Callaghan, and Uncle Paul Gordon

Abstract The aim of this chapter is to present an alternate approach to Indigenous health that is built on Ancient Indigenous Wisdoms that take into account the complex interdependency between humans and nature. The chapter first presents an overview of Indigenous commitment to nature, highlighting the broader holistic focus beyond the absence of disease. In recognition of the fact that there are many different Indigenous wisdoms, the second part of the chapter presents an example of how the Ancient Wisdoms of Australian Indigenous people can be applied to assist in providing healthcare with and for (rather than at or about) Australian Indigenous people. The chapter concludes with a discussion of the potential for a paradigm change to incorporate these wisdoms to improve Indigenous health.

11.1 Introduction

Indigenous people throughout the world have distinct cultures, yet each shares the common characteristic of a profound, purposeful relationship with the natural world. Indigenous approaches are built on the principles of complex interdependency between humans and nature. This biophilia approach can be variously termed 'connection to Country' (Kingsley et al. 2013) or 'relational reciprocity' with Country (Wall-Kimmerer 2013; Spillman et al. 2022, 2023). Historically, Indigenous people have accepted and embraced their role as guardians and custodians of ancestral lands, waterways, animals, plants, and natural resources, and many still do.

D. Vindigni OAM (✉)
STEM College, RMIT University, Melbourne, VIC, Australia
e-mail: dein.vindigni@rmit.edu.au

U. P. Callaghan · U. P. Gordon
University of New England, Armidale, NSW, Australia

S. Jones, D. Vindigni OAM (eds.), *Health and Healthcare in Complexity*,
https://doi.org/10.1007/978-981-96-0515-6_11

However, due to colonization and colonialism, this is no longer the case in all communities and for all Indigenous peoples as many Indigenous people no longer accept and embrace their role (Spillman et al. 2022, 2023).

Despite the commonalities of Indigenous people throughout the world, Uncle Paul Gordon cautions us not to reify the race-based binary notion of Indigenous/non-Indigenous as such thinking is unhelpful for a variety of reasons. Firstly, it is homogenizing, potentially leading to and reinforcing stereotyping. Secondly, the question of what 'Indigenous' means is contentious and contested. Uncle Paul Gordon does not see Indigenous identity as being connected to blood descent. Indeed, the word 'Indigenous' is derived from the Latin root meaning "native, born in a country" (https://en.wiktionary.org/wiki/indigenous) which suggests that every human is Indigenous to country somewhere. Uncle Paul Gordon makes it clear that 'Ancient Indigenous Wisdom' does not imply that all contemporary Indigenous-identifying peoples still know or live by such wisdom, whereas a growing number of non-Indigenous-identifying people do:

> Being Aboriginal is not the colour of your skin but your connection and responsibility to Country and all things in nature. It is about your connection to trees, birds, rivers, rocks and stars. It isn't about how you look. It is isn't even about your bloodline. It is about something unseen, deep inside you. (Callaghan and Gordon 2022, p, xv)

The biophilia approach acknowledges the transformation of ecosystems' energy as complex interactions between biological organisms, social beings, and the environment (Bubolz and Sontag 2009). Traditional Indigenous commitment to nature has led to criticism of the negative (Western) human impact on the health of the biosphere. This has led Buse et al. (2018, p. 420) to describe what the world is experiencing as "a new geological epoch of our own making, the Anthropocene." In contrast, the traditional, Indigenous approach is described as an "exemplar demonstrating rapid and ongoing developments in Indigenous leadership and governance for the ecological dimensions of health in relation to other social, cultural, historical and political determinants" (Buse et al. 2018, p. 422). Karulkiyalu,[1] Gordon, and Spillman (2021, p. 216) stated:

> For Indigenous peoples, everything, including humans, belongs to Country… in this way, the phrase 'custodian for Country' is more meaningful than the more conventional western phrase, 'traditional owner.'

As ancestral custodians of the land and its food, water, fibers, and medicines for millennia, Indigenous people and others connected to the land practice a holistic, integrated approach to caring for all of creation to sustain family and community throughout the generations (Langton et al. 2014).

The importance of understanding the connection between all things is highlighted by Uncle Paul Callaghan:

> Western science likes to view the world in neat identifiable segments. In our way, we are not separate at all. We are all part of the one thing. Animals, plants, humans, the earth, the waters,

[1] Karulkiyalu Country is identified as the primary author of the article.

> the sky. We are all one. We therefore need to care for all things. We need to care for each other. When we hurt one thing, we hurt the entirety. When we hurt another person we hurt ourselves.

The understanding of connection has contributed enormously to learnings of how to improve the health and well-being of all people (Viscogliosi et al. 2020). It has long been argued that there is much to learn from Indigenous people to improve their health through greater acknowledgement of the impact of their role as traditional custodians of ancestral lands (Stephens et al. 2006; Fogarty et al. 2023). In the words attributed to Chief Seattle:

> The air is precious to the red man…for all thing breath share the same breath—the beast, the trees, the man, they all share the same breath…. What is man without the beasts? If all the beasts were gone, men would die from a great loneliness of spirit. For whatever happens to the beasts, soon happens to man. All things are connected…. Whatever befalls the earth befalls the sons of the earth.

The ancient Indigenous paradigm takes into account the interconnected state of spiritual, communal, and ecosystem equilibrium and well-being (Bristow et al. 2003). Despite cultural differences between Indigenous people from different countries, many common elements, such as reverence for and custodianship of ancestral lands and acknowledgment of the connectedness of all living things, are shared. This was highlighted by the acclaimed scientist and environmentalist David Suzuki (1993), who urged Westerners to recognize the importance of the interconnectedness of all life-forms:

> ... rediscovering our kin, the other animals and plants with whom we share this planet. We are related to them through our DNA and evolution. To know our kin is to come to love and cherish them. (Suzuki 1993, p. xxx)

In so saying, Suzuki warned against the continuation of actions that are leading to the destruction of Indigenous people:

> The destruction of Indigenous people is now occurring with frightening speed. Once these people have disappeared, their body of priceless thought and knowledge, painstakingly acquired over thousands of years, will disappear forever. (Suzuki 1993, p. xxxv)

Callaghan and Gordon (2014, 2022) argued that despite the disappearance of much knowledge, the Lore for Country (that they term Earthkin) will remain with Country and reside within Indigenous Elders who have personal experiences accessing old stories for Country (Lore).

11.2 Traditional Indigenous Approaches to Health

Indigenous medicines have been used for centuries by traditional healers who bring an intimate understanding of their healing properties and their ability to promote the health and well-being of communities (Stephens et al. 2006; Redvers and Blondin 2020; De Wet et al. 2016; Fogarty et al. 2023). Blair and Collins-Gearing (2017) describe Indigenous people's profound interconnectedness with the world and the importance of listening to and learning from nature as steps to knowings. Indigenous people throughout the world have contributed enormously to knowledge of how to improve the health and well-being of all people (Viscogliosi et al. 2020; Yunkaporta 2023). In the words of an Elder Grandmother of the Cree Nation:

> Strengths are about a way of being through Relationships with ourselves, people, the land, ancestors and all beings; these connections are a reflection and extension of self. These strengths are lived through actions in the Circle as opportunities to engage, learn, connect and re-engage when we lose our way. Strengths are directed at the Common Good, for the benefit of all, and validated in our Accountability to the common good of all beings. We share our strengths with Humility and Respect, and Without Fear. This is practiced as Helping and understood as a Present opportunity. We need to understand and share strengths as Gifts, and it is our Responsibility to keep that vibration in our hearts. (Doreen Spence, Saddle Lake Cree Nation)

This has led to a change in approach to Indigenous health, away from emphasizing the negative impact of colonialization, to a focus on how to use Ancient Indigenous Wisdoms to improve Indigenous health. Indigenous approaches form the basis for what has been termed an Indigenous strengths-based[2] approach to healthcare that recognizes the distinguished capacities and capabilities of Indigenous peoples (Rigney 2017). Fogarty et al. (2023) spoke of an emerging trend toward strengths-based approaches, which demonstrate promising health outcomes for Aboriginal communities and service providers. They argued that an Indigenous strengths-based approach highlights the strengths and richness of Indigenous communities and cultures. They contrasted this with Western research and media reports of Indigenous health that have historically focused on deficit discourses that highlight pathology, risky behaviors, and dysfunctional stereotypes assumed to be inherent in Aboriginal communities (Reading and Nowgesic 2002; Halpern 2015; AHRC 2023). In contrast, Fogarty et al. (2023) argued for more indigenist research that emphasizes the value of collaborative projects and research that are carried out with and for, rather than at or about, Indigenous people. Indigenist approaches give voice to the voiceless and thereby challenge the dominance of Western-orientated discourse. This includes the resilience, ingenuity, and adaptability of Indigenous communities to not only survive but to thrive in complex, ever-changing geographical and sociocultural landscapes.

11.3 Traditional Indigenous Wisdoms and Indigenous Health

Indigenous wisdoms are a product of their cultures, which in turn are built on sociocultural decision systems that are grounded in community discussion; iteration with other animals, plants, and life-forms in the ecosystem; and deep spiritual reflection.

---

[2] Note: The term "strengths-based approach" is used in other sections of this book to refer to a forward-looking, rather than backward-looking, approach; consequently, we have used the term "Indigenous strengths-based approach" to differentiate the use in this sense.

They are shown in the embedding of community-specific cultural and ceremonial practices to strengthen relationships with country and community and promote healing (Archibald 2006). This has resulted in a plethora of examples of Indigenous customs, traditions, and kinship systems that continue to exist in communities alongside attempts to reclaim and preserve Indigenous cultures. Although most initiatives start with a broad-based focus on the value of learning from, and conducting respectful and meaningful consultation with, Indigenous Elders (Evolve Communities 2024; Abercrombie 2020). An example of Australian Indigenous wisdoms relating to Indigenous health is presented below. This is taken from the writing of one Indigenous Elder of an Aboriginal language group[3] (Kakkib Li'Dthia Warrawee'a 2000), who believes that the poor health of Indigenous Australians in today's world can be traced to spiritual, environmental, and social degradation. While acknowledging the over 700 nations or language groups of Australian Indigenous groups that existed before colonization, the Indigenous Elder identifies four common, essential philosophies (or tenets) that are shared throughout many language groups: Aildt, Adtomon, Dtwongdtyen, and Linj'dta (Kakkib Li'Dthia Warrawee'a 2002).

1. Aildt: Everything is One

The first tenet, Aidlt, can be loosely translated into English as "one spirit – all things" (Kakkib Li'Dthia Warrawee'a 2002, p. 25). Kakkib Li'Dthia Warrawee'a explains that everything, tangible and intangible, springs from the Creator; we are all One. The implication is that a holistic approach to health must address the mind, body, spirit, social, and environmental well-being of the individual and the Community. This view contrasts with the Western monotheistic view, which distinguishes between animate (with a spirit) and inanimate beings.

2. Adtomon: Truth is the path

The second tenet, Adtomon, can be loosely translated into English as "follow the path of truth-honour and be honoured: live according to the laws of nature; and be true to yourself" (Kakkib Li'Dthia Warrawee'a 2002, p. 27). Kakkib Li'Dthia Warrawee'a explains that it doesn't matters if people's truths differ, as long as one's truth abides by the laws of nature to which one is true. The implication for health is that when individuals lose track of their truth, disease may occur.

3. Dtwongdtyen: A varied perspective is the key to perception

The third tenet, Dtwongdtyen, can be loosely translated into English as "to see things from varied viewpoints and different perspectives" (Li'Dthia Warrawee'a 2002, p. 27). The implication is that there is need to see and approach health from many perspectives.

[3] Indigenous Elders are respected as the most valued knowledge-holders who, through rigorous lifelong ceremonial training and practice, hold expert knowledge of Indigenous ways of being and knowing. This example is of a senior Elder and teacher of the Ya-idt'midtung, from Northeastern Victoria and the Kosciuszko region of NSW, Australia.

4. Linj'dta: Now is the moment of your being

The fourth tenet, Linj'dta, can be loosely translated into "one must live in 'the present', for now is the moment of our being" (Kakkib Li'Dthia Warrawee'a 2002, p. 33–34). The implication is the need to be present in the moment rather than the past, as to dwell in the past is more likely to lead to depression and insecurities and to focus on the future is to be consumed by the unknown and invite fears and anxieties to enter one's being.

Uncle Paul Gordon warns us that this doesn't mean the past should be ignored (Callaghan and Gordon 2022, pp. 213–214):

> Your past is important. If you don't know your past, if you don't know your story, if you don't know where you come from, then you will be sitting in the present moment lost…If I don't have that story of my past, I can't go back, and if there are things from the past hurting me, holding me down, affecting my self-esteem, I might end up angry or I might end up being sad. I can't change my past but I can address it.

The conclusion from these tenets is that Indigenous Australians need to reclaim their Ancient Wisdoms that were lost due to colonization. In a lecture to university students in 2003, Kakkib Li'Dthia Warrawee'a stated:

> If Aboriginal people lose their culture, their language and their heritage, they lose their self-esteem and often, with it, their will to live. If you lose your will to live, no medicine, doctor or health clinic will keep you alive. The path forward for us requires acknowledging and reaffirming the giftedness of all people, particularly the wisdom of the ancients. (Personal notes of attendee at the lecture)

11.4 Application of Ancient Indigenous Wisdoms to Improve Indigenous Health

There are promising examples of the integration of traditional, Indigenous approaches into mainstream healthcare. In New Zealand, a pioneering model of healthcare has been adopted that aims to embed the engagement and involvement of the Indigenous (Māori) population in health initiatives to provide more equitable access for Māori (Panesar et al. 2021). This approach is built on "a shared mental model and mutual understanding of the attitudes and barriers towards health improvement and heath equity" (Panesar et al. 2021, p. 83). Complementing this health focus has been an exploration of a 'radical ecosystem' of collective leadership built on the Māori concept of biofilia that is described as "grounded in an animated world of affection between humans and cosmos, where we are evolving together – entwined in sacred kinship" (Spiller et al. 2020, p. 518). This radical ecosystem leadership emphasizes the need to encourage (1) networks of dynamic relationships between individuals and collectives, (2) identification and adherence to a knowledge code to hold the dynamic networks together, and (3) encouragement of "ties of affection that bind people to each other, to place and ecologies and ensure that leadership is honouring the knowledge code" (Spiller et al. 2020, p. 519).

In Australia, a National Strategic Framework for Aboriginal and Torres Strait Islander (ATSI) Peoples' Mental Health and Social and Emotional Wellbeing (National Strategic Framework 2023) aims at improving the mental health and social and emotional well-being of Indigenous Australians. This framework is based on a holistic model of social and emotional well-being previously described by Gee et al. (2014). It adopts a self-determination approach that places the individual self at its center, connected synergistically to the political, social, and historical environment, through the body, mind, emotions, family and kinship, Community, spirit, spirituality and ancestors, Country, and culture. These domains give Aboriginal and Torres Strait Islander peoples an optimal foundation to support a strong and positive sense of belonging and collective identity conducive to health through three elements:

(i) Cultural determinants of health which include culture and cultural identity, and which involves a living relationship with ancestors the spiritual aspects of existence and connection to Country and language. This can influence decisions about seeking health services, acceptance of and compliance with treatment, and success of prevention and health-promotion strategies.
(ii) Individual and Community control over one's physical environment, autonomy, dignity, and self-respect and a perception of fair and just treatment (Calma et al. 2017).
(iii) Social determinants of health, including education and unemployment, and responses to a broader range of problems resulting from historical determinants such as colonization and its intergenerational legacies: grief and loss, trauma and abuse, violence, removal from family and cultural dislocation, substance abuse, racism and discrimination, and social disadvantage.

Additionally, a Family Wellbeing Empowerment (FWA) program developed in the early 1990s has been successfully adapted into many Indigenous communities throughout Australia (Whiteside et al. 2014). The program is focused on the aim of "empowering individuals, families, organisations and communities to improve their condition" (Whiteside et al. 2014, p. vii). It adopts a holistic, integrated approach to healthcare that is sensitive and responsive to the role of physical, mental, emotional, and spiritual needs of individuals, their families, and their Community. This is achieved by emphasizing "building the individual's and community's capacity to transform and take greater control of their own processes in their lives" (Whiteside et al. 2014, p. 43). The model for the program incorporates several interconnected elements of empowerment: beliefs and attitudes, skills and knowledge, agency and outcomes, and their interaction with the broader social environment. The model has been assessed as resonating strongly with Aboriginal understandings of social and emotional well-being and provides a practical framework for action (Whiteside et al. 2014, p. vii). These integrated principles are used to guide regular (usually weekly) workshops that help participants to acquire and affirm the knowledge, skills, and confidence required to "build their capacity to transform and take greater control of their own processes for change" (Whiteside et al. 2014). FWAs are usually conducted in culturally safe and inclusive community centers and often include a range of Community representatives such as Elders, teachers, parents, and mainstream health workers and traditional healers, as well as Community leaders. Some notable outcomes of the program include participants "healing from past abuse, reducing their alcohol consumption, taking on new challenges in relation to education and employment and establishing more harmonious relationships" (Whiteside et al. 2014, p. 43).

11.5 Discussion

An important implication of acquiring a greater understanding of, and adherence to, Ancient Indigenous Wisdoms is a more holistic, integrated approach to healthcare that takes into account the complex interactions between humans and nature. Adoption of such an approach also has implications for Western approaches to health and healthcare. Attena (2016) contrasts the Indigenous approach with the Western (Cartesian science) approach to healthcare, which has led to healthcare being directed at the patient, rather than proactively involving and empowering the person to participate in their own care.

At a time when dominant Western cultures suffer from an epidemic of stress and disconnection on so many levels, Ancient Indigenous Wisdoms challenge us to rediscover meaning and purpose in personal and community relationships and connection to mother nature (Jewson 2009). This is bringing Indigenous peoples' approach to well-being closer to the aspirational Western paradigm of a holistic approach to health that goes beyond the original narrower focus on health as the absence of disease. It is in keeping with increasing widespread acknowledgement of healthcare as a complex system characterized by the following:

> self-organizing, adaptive, emergent, comprised of a large number of elements, autopoietic, nonlinear, dynamic, network-like in structure, open-ended with fuzzy boundaries, interdependent, agent-based, evolving, chaotic, comprised of feedback loops, historical, nodes within a larger network of systems, environmentally impacted, etc. … Together and in isolation, the characteristics of a complex system not only describe what it is; they explain how it works. (Castellani et al. 2015, p. 3)[4]

11.6 Summary

An understanding, of and adherence, to the implications of Ancient Indigenous Wisdoms has a range of implications for how the health and healthcare of Indigenous people is perceived and implemented. The Ancient Wisdoms enable a return to a focus on the biophilia, in which Indigenous approaches to healthcare are built on the

[4] Further exploration is the potential conjoining of the Indigenous paradigm and the Western paradigm discussed in Chap. 13.

principles of complex interdependency between humans and nature. These implications are discussed in the next chapter.

References

Abercrombie J (2020) Mental Well-being of Aboriginal Adults in Canada: Intergenerational impact of Attending Residential Schools. Åbo Akademi University

Archibald L (2006) Decolonization and healing: indigenous experiences in the United States, New Zealand, Australia and Greenland. Aboriginal Healing Foundation, Ottawa

Attena F (2016) Limitations of Western Medicine and Models of Integration Between Medical Systems. J Altern Complement Med 22(5):343. Review Articles, normal Published Online: https://doi.org/10.1089/acm.2015.0381

Australian Human Rights Commission (AHRC) (2023) Racism: it stops with me. Available from: https://itstopswithme.humanrights.gov.au/resourcehub

Blair N, Collins-Gearing B (2017) Reflective practice: ancient wisdom and practice—Australian indigenous reflections in teacher education through shared storying. In: Reflective theory and practice in teacher education. Springer, pp 63–83

Bristow F, Nettleton C, Stephens C, Mijlof I, Iona J, Hart T, McCausland C (2003) Utz Wachil

Bubolz MM, Sontag MS (2009) Chapter 1: Human ecology theory. In: Boss P, Doherty WJ, LaRossa WR, Steinmetz SK (eds) Sourcebook of family theories and methods. Springer, Boston MA, pp 419–450

Buse CG, Oestreicher JS, Ellis NR, Patrick R, Brisbois B, Jenkins AP, McKellar K, Kingsley J, Gislason M, Galway L, McFarlane RA (2018) Public health guide to field developments linking ecosystems, environments and health in the Anthropocene. J Epidemiol Community Health 72(5):420–425

Callaghan P, Gordon P (2022) The dreaming path: Indigenous thinking to change your life. Pantera Press

Callaghan, Paul with Uncle Gordon P (2014) Iridescence: finding your colours and living your story. MoshPit Publishing, Hazelwood, NSW

Calma T, Dudgeon P, Bray A (2017) Aboriginal and Torres Strait islander social and emotional wellbeing and mental health. Aust Psychol 52(4):255–260

Castellani B, Rjaram R, Buckwalter JG et al (2015) Place and health as complex systems: a case-study and empirical test, SpringerBriefs in Public Health. Springer. https://doi.org/10.1007/978-3-319-09734-3

De Wet H, Ramulondi M, Ngcobo ZN (2016) The use of indigenous medicine for the treatment of hypertension by a rural community in northern Maputaland, South Africa. S Afr J Bot 103:78–88

Evolve Communities, https://www.evolves.com.au/impact-colonisation-indigenous-australians/. Accessed 20 Jan 2024

Fogarty W, Lovell M, Langenberg J, Heron MJ (2023) Deficit discourse and strengths-based approaches: changing the narrative of Aboriginal and Torres Strait Islander Health and Wellbeing 2018. Available from: https://rb.gy/oz2s5

Gee G, Dudgeon P, Schultz C, Hart A, Kelly, K (2014) Aboriginal and Torres Strait Islander social and emotional wellbeing. Working together: Aboriginal and Torres Strait Islander mental health and wellbeing principles and practice, 2: 55–68. Australian Government Department of the Prime Minister and Cabinet

Halpern D (2015) Inside the nudge unit. Ebury Publishing, London

Hands on Health-About us https://hoha.org.au/about-us/2022

Jewson ND (2009) The disappearance of the sick-man from medical cosmology, 1770–1870. International. J Epidemiol 38(3):622–633

Kakkib Li'Dthia Warrawee'a (2000) An aboriginal perspective on holistic health. Diver Nat Complement Health 2(2):2–9

Kakkib li'Dthia Warrawee'a (2002) There once was a tree called Deru / Kakkib li'Dthia Warrawee'a, Thorsons Pymble, N.S.W

Kakkib Li'Dthia Warrawee'a (2003) Wisdom, knowledge, information: have we lost our way in our understanding and practice of medicine? Lecture. RMIT University, Melbourne, City Campus Thursday 21 August

Karulkiyalu, Country, Gordon P, Spillman D (2021) Embracing country as teacher in outdoor and environmental education. In Thomas G, Dyment J, Prince H (eds.) Outdoor environmental education in higher education, (9): 215–224. Springer

Kingsley J, Townsend M, Henderson-Wilson C, Bolam B (2013) Developing an exploratory framework linking Australian aboriginal peoples' connection to country and concepts of wellbeing. Int J Environ Res Public Health 10(2):678–698

Langton M, Palmer L, Rhea ZM (2014) Community-oriented protected areas for indigenous peoples and local communities. In: Indigenous peoples, national parks, and protected areas: A new paradigm linking conservation, culture, and rights. The University of Arizona Press, p 84

National Strategic Framework for Aboriginal and Torres Strait Islander Peoples' Mental Health and Social and Emotional Wellbeing 2017–2023 (2023) National Indigenous Australians Agency. Available at: https://www.niaa.gov.au/resource-centre/indigenous-affairs/national-strategic-framework-mental-health-social-emotional-wellbeing-2017-23. Accessed 17 Feb 2024

Panesar D, Rahiri JL, Koea J (2021) Indigenous Health Leadership: A Kaupapa Māori Perspective from Aotearoa–New Zealand. BMJ Leader 5(2):83

Reading J, Nowgesic E (2002) Improving the health of future generations: the Canadian institutes of health research institute of Aboriginal peoples' health. Am J Public Health 92(9):1396-1400.s

Redvers N, Blondin BS (2020) Traditional indigenous medicine in North America: a scoping review. PLoS One 15(8):e0237531

Rigney LI (2017) Indigenist research and aboriginal Australia. In: Indigenous peoples' wisdom and power. Routledge, pp 32–48

Spiller C, Maunganui Wolfgramm R, Henry E, Pouwhare R (2020) Paradigm warriors: advancing a radical ecosystems view of collective leadership from an Indigenous Māori perspective. Hum Relat 73(4):516–543

Spillman D, Wilson B, Nixon M, McKinnon K (2022) Reinvigorating country as teacher in Australian schooling: beginning with school teacher's direct experiences, 'relating with country'. Curric Perspect 43:13. https://doi.org/10.1007/s41297-022-00176-6

Spillman D, Wilson B, Nixon M, McKinnon K (2023) New localism' in Australian schools: Country as Teacher as a critical pedagogy of place. Curric Perspect 43:103. https://doi.org/10.1007/s41297-023-00201-2

Stephens C, Porter J, Nettleton C, Willis R (2006) Disappearing, displaced, and undervalued: a call to action for Indigenous health worldwide. Lancet 367(9527):2019–2028

Suzuki D (1993) Wisdom of the elders: sacred native stories of nature. BoD–Books on Demand

Viscogliosi C, Asselin H, Basile S, Borwick K, Couturier Y, Drolet MJ, Levasseur M (2020) Importance of Indigenous elders' contributions to individual and community wellness: results from a scoping review on social participation and intergenerational solidarity. Can J Public Health 111:667–681

Wall-Kimmerer R (2013) Braiding sweetgrass: Indigenous wisdom, scientific knowledge and the teachings of plants. Penguin

Whiteside M, Tsey K, Cadet-James Y, McCalman J (2014) Promoting aboriginal health: the family wellbeing empowerment approach. Springer Science and Business Media

Yunkaporta T (2023) Sand talk: how indigenous thinking can save the world. Naarm (Melbourne) Wurundjeri Country: Text Publishing, The Text Publishing Company

Chapter 12
An Ancient Indigenous Wisdoms Framework

Dein Vindigni OAM, Uncle Paul Callaghan, and Uncle Paul Gordon

Abstract The aim of this chapter is to present a framework for Indigenous health based in acknowledgment of biophilia (commitment to the fundamental principle of the importance of nature) and the Ancient Wisdoms of Indigenous Elders (both discussed in the previous chapter). The chapter first discusses a respectful appreciation and deeper understanding of Indigenous culture before presenting a reinterpretation of the Old people's knowledge and wisdom for contemporary society through six Ls (Lore, Love, Look, Listen, Learn, Lead [or Leave alone]).

12.1 Introduction

The World Health Organization (WHO) (2017) states that health is a human right for all. In its Declaration on the Rights of Indigenous Peoples, the United Nations (UNDRIP) outlines 'minimum standards for the survival, dignity, and well-being of the Indigenous peoples of the world' (UN 2007, p. 28). This reflects on the importance of protecting culturally based strengths, including the right to self-determination and to address inequity. Action to implement these commitments varies between countries. In Canada, the guiding framework for the Truth and Reconciliation Commission (TRC 2015) supports change that stresses the importance of reclaiming cultural strengths and recognizing deep-seated capacities for resilience, healing, and wellness in individuals, families, and communities (Kennedy et al. 2022). In Australia, this is supported through a focus on cultural security and

D. Vindigni OAM (✉)
STEM College, RMIT University, Melbourne, VIC, Australia
e-mail: dein.vindigni@rmit.edu.au

U. P. Callaghan · U. P. Gordon
University of New England, Armidale, NSW, Australia

S. Jones, D. Vindigni OAM (eds.), *Health and Healthcare in Complexity*,
https://doi.org/10.1007/978-981-96-0515-6_12

the action that stresses the importance of commitment that health systems will not compromise the cultural rights, values, views, and expectations of Indigenous peoples, as a rights-based policy commitment to engaging with cultural humility and facilitating culturally safe and quality healthcare (Lock et al. 2019).

12.2 Culture, Cultural Competence, and Indigenous Thinking

Culture and cultural competence in Indigenous thinking is composed of many elements: cultural awareness, cultural sensitivity, and cultural humility. Cultural awareness has been defined as the:

> process of conducting a self-examination of one's assumptions and biases (both conscious and unconscious) towards other cultures and the in-depth exploration of one's cultural and professional background. It involves being aware of the existence of discrimination, prejudice, and exclusionary practices in healthcare delivery. (Prehn et al. 2021, p. 29)

Cultural sensitivity involves employing one's knowledge, consideration, understanding, respect, and tailoring after realizing awareness of self and others and encountering a diverse group or individual (Foronda 2008).

Cultural humility requires deeper reflective, and empathic exchanges. This involves:

> entering a healthy relationship with another person with the intention of honouring their beliefs, customs, and values, and entails an ongoing process of self-exploration and self-critique combined with a willingness to learn from others'. (Stubbe 2020, p. 49)

Tervalon and Murray-Garcia (1998) describe cultural humility as a "lifelong process of self-reflection and self-critique whereby the individual not only learns about another's culture but starts with an examination of her/his own beliefs and cultural identities" (Tervalon and Murray-Garcia 1998, p. 117). It is claimed that adopting cultural humility which recognizes "the limits of one's knowledge and appreciating others' intellectual strengths" (Porter and Schumann 2018, p. 139) can help facilitate strong working alliances between therapists and diverse clients, leading to better outcomes (Yeager and Bauer-Wu 2013). Embracing cultural humility encourages respect for Indigenous perspectives as:

> a process of self-reflection to understand personal and systemic biases and to develop and maintain respectful processes and relationships based on mutual trust. Cultural humility involves humbly acknowledging oneself as a learner when it comes to understanding another's experience. (Phelan 2021, p. 32)

Cultural competence is seen as a necessary condition for working effectively with diverse patients in healthcare. This is based on an assumption that the more knowledge one has about another culture, the greater their competence in engaging with colleagues professionally (Phelan 2021, p. 32).

In addition to cultural competence, cultural safety is seen as necessary to provide a safe environment for Indigenous people. Cultural safety is described as:

an environment that is safe for people: where there is no assault, challenge or denial of their identity, of who they are and what they need. It is about shared respect, shared meaning, shared knowledge, and experience of learning, living and working together with dignity and truly listening. (Williams 1999, p. 213)

Maori Elders have expressed their belief that:

ensuring the inclusion of Indigenous and non-Indigenous knowledge in contemporary health developments not only underpins Indigenous sustainability and resilience, it also provides Indigenous people with a platform to participate in national and global developments in ways that can build the sustainability and resilience of Indigenous and non-Indigenous peoples together. (Chant 2013, pg. 111-1 V)

An example of how to respectfully engage with Indigenous people in Australia is embedded in Uncle Paul Gordon's teachings of the 6Ls (Lore, Love, Look, Listen, Learn, Lead [or Leave Alone]) (Callaghan and Gordon 2014). The Australian Indigenous 6Ls are a reinterpretation of the Old People's knowledge and wisdom for contemporary society. These 6Ls align with other Indigenous teachings such as Dadirri (an Aboriginal word shared by Aunty Miriam Rose Ungunmerr-Baumann AM from the Ngan'gikurunggurr and Ngen'giwumirri languages of the Aboriginal peoples of the Daly River region, Northern Territory, Australia) that can be loosely translated into English as 'inner deep listening and quiet, still awareness and waiting' (Ungunmerr 2017, p. 14).

12.3 The 6Ls of Australian Indigenous Wisdoms

In Australia, six key principles for engaging with Indigenous communities were developed by one of the authors of this chapter, Uncle Paul Gordon (Karulkiyalu et al. 2021). They are used as a teaching and learning process to enact Indigenous ways of knowing, being, and doing as follows.

12.3.1 Lore

Indigenous Australians have a complex system of *lore* that existed long before the establishment of British *law* in Australia or other colonies. For Indigenous people, Lore preserves and shares the values, ancient knowledge, and wisdom required to exist in harmony with each other and all of creation (Rose 2011; Karulkiyalu et al. 2021):

The Lore [is] an English word which can be considered to mean the traditional knowledge passed on from generation to generation (through song, story, sites and dance) that guides all aspects of our life. The traditional wording that captures the concept of the Lore differs across the continent, as can interpretations of its meaning; however, in essence, the Lore states we all have a responsibility to care for our place and all things in our place. (Callaghan and Gordon 2022, p. 9)

Although Lore may be taught by different stories in different Communities, the values are the same. Understanding and respecting local Lore and traditions when engaging with Aboriginal people from other language groups is critically important for developing and maintaining respectful, collaborative partnerships. Lore, which is the foundation for all that we do or don't do, is explained by Karulkiyalu Country, Gordon, and Spillman (2021, p. 218): "it becomes the motivation for us to expend energy to continue learning about Country and how to look after particular Earth-kin Country."

12.3.2 Love

The second important L is Love and good intentions to motivate all exchanges and relationships which are themselves based in Lore and a love of the Lore. This is important in the history of Indigenous, Western relations which include many examples of well-intentioned missionaries motivated by 'love' but who often intentionally disregarded the first principle of Indigenous Lore, with damaging and even disastrous consequences:

> The first thing we have to know before we can help anybody is their story. We have to know the Lore relating to their story; that is, we have to know the rules, responsibilities and obligations relating to their story. Once we know their story, then we can act in love because we will respect their story and make sure what we do fits in with that story. What we do will be right. (Callaghan and Gordon 2022, p. 91)

There are many examples of restrictions, or removing, of Indigenous spiritual and cultural practices such as song, dance, ceremonial gatherings, language, hunting and gathering, traditional foods, and medicines that were not in accord with Western views. These actions were part of a government commitment to Aboriginal assimilation, captured in 1953 in the following statement by newly appointed federal Minister for Territories, Paul Hasluck, that "Assimilation means, in practical terms, that in the course of time, it is expected that all persons of aboriginal blood and mixed blood in Australia will live like the white Australians do" (Hasluck 1953, p. 16). This policy of assimilation led to disconnecting Aboriginal people from Country, kinship and culture with the widespread and longstanding destruction that followed.

12.3.3 Look

The third L is Look. Uncle Paul Gordon explains the importance of looking as follows (Callaghan and Gordon 2014, pp. 46–47):

> Most of us are aware of the notion of actively listening, but actively watching is also important. To train our eyes to actively watch, the Old People tell us how important it is to go and sit in the bush or forest and just look. We are taught to sit for hours and, if possible, days on our own and just watch what is around us… By actively looking you will notice a great deal and possibly achieve some surprising insights. You might have insights about patience, hidden beauty, persistence, hope, movement, trust, change, diversity, unity and wonderment. All of this by being quiet and looking.

To look provides an opportunity to observe and begin to appreciate what practices are acceptable and non-acceptable in various Community settings. These cultural practices and traditions may vary from Community to Community and inform more culturally sensitive responses and interactions with people from other communities. Karulkiyalu Country, Gordon, and Spillman (2021, p. 218) explain that Looking and Listening attentively will awaken and enhance our "perceptive capabilities to notice and observe Earth-Kin."

12.3.4 Listen

The fourth L is Listen. To listen, particularly deeply and patiently, is centrally important in all exchanges with Aboriginal people and ideally between all people (Callaghan and Gordon 2014, p. 46):

> The way we learn about people's stories is by looking and listening. Sitting with one another; listening to one another, looking at what the Old People are showing us, looking at what the land is showing us, what the animals are showing us, listening to the land, watching the land, we grow by looking and listening.

Looking and Listening patiently and respectfully allows others to more fully tell their story as a step toward building and sustaining relationships of trust and goodwill. A common message in Aboriginal spirituality is the importance of listening to and learning from each other with a deep sense of humility, patience, mutual respect, and inclusion wherever we come from or whatever our beliefs are. Vindigni (2004, p. 17) references a reflection of the late Dr. Puggy Hunter in an address to ear, nose, and throat specialists:

> You white people keep telling us Aboriginals that we have ear problems. You keep showing us the graphs and the research. You know, I think you mob are the ones with ear problems. We keep saying the same things and you don't seem to hear.

This message is reinforced by the late Uncle Neville Buchanan who Vindigni (2004, p. 17) reports as often stating, "the Creator gave us two ears and one mouth so that we could listen twice and speak once," together with Uncle Paul Gordon who has stated "we must share the gifts of creation more fairly, nurture each other and the land which, like an umbilical cord, sustains us."

12.3.5 Learn

The fifth L is to Learn. We look and listen in order to gain knowledge so we can better connect with what is around us. If we connect with what is around us, we learn. If we learn, we grow. If we grow, we find meaning. If we find meaning, we have purpose. If we have purpose, we are better able to fulfil our potential. If we fulfil our potential, we find contentment (Callaghan and Gordon 2022, pp. 137–138). To learn is ultimately dependent on having the cultural respect, humility, and patience to quietly absorb and reflect upon the knowledge and wisdom that comes from these earlier steps of respect for and understanding of the wisdom of Elders and Community. This is in keeping with a quote from Grandmother Doreen from Saddle Lake Cree Nation, repeated in Kennedy et al. (2022, p. 425) that emphasizes the importance of:

> starting where people are at and bringing them forward with love and respect to learn our ways for reconciliation… we would never have a university without a library, and Elders are the library for Indigenous peoples.

12.3.6 Lead [or Leave Alone]

The final L important to Indigenous Australians is to Lead. In traditional settings, to lead is to achieve the best outcomes for all involved in both emerging and established relationships with people and Country. This occurs once all the other Ls have been considered. However, in some cases, once all 6Ls have been considered, it may be more prudent and even necessary to simply leave the situation alone if positive and productive outcomes already exist. Karulkiyalu Country, Gordon, and Spillman (2021, p. 218) state that this has led to recommendation for a:

> rebalancing of teaching and learning approaches– away from those that prioritise human-centred, rational knowledge, towards more locally-oriented, ecocentric approaches that utilize and rebalance all our ways of knowing, being and doing and that focus on restoring ecological (including human) balance and wellbeing.

12.4 Discussion

Examples of the integration of traditional, Indigenous approaches into mainstream Western educational approaches exist in Indigenous communities throughout the world. In Canada, the emphasis has been on the value of adopting co-learning and meaningful consultation with Indigenous Canadian Elders to explore how social innovation through co-learning and meaningful consultation raises opportunities for positive disruption that challenges entrenched traditional colonial educational perspectives (Kennedy et al. 2023). Kennedy et al. (2022) highlight the strengths-based approaches that are present in some frameworks for Indigenous health professions education, especially in nursing and medicine. These include recognition of eight interconnected actions to support Indigenous health equity: (1) respecting Indigenous human rights, (2) respecting Indigenous knowledges and healing practices, (3) recentering power relationships, (4) revitalizing culture and collective identity, (5) cultivating individual and collective resilience, (6) advancing equity, (7) advancing self-determination, and (8) capacity building with individuals and communities (Kennedy et al. 2022, p. 430).

In New Zealand, an innovative cross-cultural education program was developed through a collaboration between local Indigenous people and childhood educators, who embraced the wisdom of the Maori Elders to care deeply for mother nature as co-habitors of the Earth (Ritchie 2014).

In Australia, the implications of Indigenous wisdoms embedded in the 6Ls has resulted in some changes for teaching and learning. Several innovative educational programs have been codesigned and co-delivered to embrace the principles and framework of a strengths-based approach. In one project, a learning program was codesigned and co-delivered by Aboriginal academics in collaboration with preservice teachers, to educate non-Indigenous people (Blair and Collins-Gearing 2017). In another project, an '8Ways pedagogical framework' was codesigned and codeveloped to help teachers to include Aboriginal perspectives. This uses Aboriginal learning techniques that focus on relational responsiveness that go beyond cultural awareness, cultural sensitivity, and even cultural responsiveness, to create a great understanding of Aboriginal ways of learning. The 8Ways pedagogical framework highlights Indigenous processes of knowledge transition: story sharing; learning maps that picture pathways of knowledge; nonverbal application of intra-personal and kinesthetic skill to thinking and learning; symbols, images, and metaphors to understand concepts and content; land links for place-based learning, linking content to local land and place; nonlinear (lateral and systems) thinking to produce innovations; deconstruction/reconstruction working from whole to parts to watch and then do; and Community links to apply learning locally for community benefit (Bangamalnha Centre 2024, https://www.8ways.online/our-protocol). Another example from Australia is a project established called Aboriginal Health in Aboriginal Hands (AHAH) that was established under the auspices of an international voluntary health organization, Hands on Health Australia (HoHA). The AHAH program was established in collaboration with Uncle Paul Gordon and further developed and implemented by Gunditjmara healer, April Clarke. It provides culturally sensitive, allied, and complementary health services to an Aboriginal Football and Netball Club. Members of the Community, Aboriginal health workers, coaches, and students of chiropractic at a major metropolitan Australian university collaborate and provide the services. This level of collaboration helps draw on the collective practical wisdom of community members to facilitate holistic, integrated approaches to healthcare that may better address the socioeconomic and cultural contributors to health. The AHAH program includes an adaptation of a Sustainable Training Treatment Employment Program (STTEP) that provides a blend of traditional, Indigenous, and Western hands-on healing approaches to community-based Indigenous healthcare which is being implemented in various communities (Vindigni et al. 2009, 2011; Stavridis 2023). This program embraces a 'whole-of-life' view that respects the concept of 'life-death-life' which presents a holistic understanding of health, though complex, ambitious, and not readily embraced or funded by conservative Western models of healthcare, arguably more successful in its outlook and application (Jackson Pulver et al. 2019).

12.5 Conclusion

This chapter has argued that to respond appropriately to improving the health and well-being of Indigenous people, a strengths-based approach that respects the self-determination of Indigenous peoples from their perspective, is needed (Askew et al. 2020). Such a strengths-based approach would incorporate the reclamation of Ancient Indigenous Wisdoms that recognize the interconnectedness between people and nature and are influenced by a traditional holistic approach to health and well-being. This approach provides an anchor upon which learnings and practices can be preserved and transmitted intergenerationally and cross-culturally to promote the health and well-being of all people.

In the words of Uncle Paul Callaghan:

> *when understood, respected and practised, the ancient traditions and learnings of lore will continue to bring hope and healing to all people and all of all of creation.*

References

Askew DA, Brady K, Mukandi B, Singh D, Sinha T, Brough M, Bond CJ (2020) Closing the gap between rhetoric and practice in strengths approaches to Indigenous public health: a qualitative study. Aust N Z J Public Health 44(2):102–105

Bangamalhanha Centre, Regional Aboriginal education team, Department of Education (2024). https://www.8ways.online/our-protocol. Western NSW. NSW Agency for Clinical Innovation

Blair N, Collins-Gearing B (2017) Reflective practice: Ancient Wisdom and Practice—Australian Indigenous reflections in teacher education through shared storying. In: Reflective theory and practice in teacher education. Springer, Singapore, pp 63–83

Callaghan P, Gordon P (2014) Iridescence: finding your colours and living your story. Moshpit Publishing, Hazelbrook

Callaghan P, Gordon P (2022) The dreaming path. Pantera, Neutral Bay

Chant L (2013) Hauora Kotahitanga. Maori health experiences as models for co-operative co-existence between indigenous and non-indigenous peoples. Doctoral dissertation ResearchSpace@ Auckland

Foronda C (2008) Cultural sensitivity: a concept analysis. J Transcult Nurs 19(3):207–212

Hasluck P (1953) Native welfare in Australia. Patterson Brokensha, Perth

Jackson Pulver L, Williams M, Fitzpatrick S (2019) Social determinants of Australia's First Peoples health: a multi-level empowerment perspective. In: Social determinants of health. Oxford University Press

Karulkiyalu, Country, Gordon P, Spillman D (2021) Embracing country as teacher in outdoor and environmental education. In Thomas G, Dyment J, Prince H (eds.) Outdoor environmental education in higher education, (9): 215–224. Springer

Kennedy A, Sehgal A, Szabo J, McGowan K, Lindstrom G, Roach P, Crowshoe L, Barnabe C (2022) Indigenous strengths-based approaches to healthcare and health professions education—recognising the value of Elders' teachings. Health Educ J 81(4):423–438. https://doi.org/10.1177/00178969221088921

Kennedy A, McGowan K, El-Hussein M (2023) Indigenous Elders' wisdom and dominionization in higher education: barriers and facilitators to decolonisation and reconciliation. Int J Incl Educ 27(1):89–106

Lock MJ, Hartz D, Martin R, et al. (2019) An aboriginal cultural safety and security framework: improving aboriginal health outcomes through culturally safe and secure mainstream healthcare governance and practice. Port Macquarie, NSW, Australia: Mid North Coast Local Health District and the Mid North Coast Aboriginal Health Authority

Phelan P (2021) Aboriginal fields of practice, edited by Bindi Bennett. Bloomsbury Publishing

Porter T, Schumann K (2018) Intellectual humility and openness to the opposing view. Self Identity 17(2):139–162

Prehn J, Krakouer J, Fernando T, Phelan P, Russ-Smith J, Wheeler A (2021) Aboriginal fields of practice. Bloomsbury Publishing

Ritchie J (2014) Learning from the wisdom of elders. In: Research in early childhood education for sustainability: International perspectives and provocations. Routledge, pp 49–60

Rose DB (2011) Wild dog dreaming: love and extinction. University of Virginia Press

Stavridis S (2023) An evaluation of the factors affecting the success of an Indigenous Community based healthcare clinic: The Hands on Health Australia's Community Clinic, and its program—Aboriginal Health in Aboriginal Hands, at the Fitzroy Stars Football and Netball Club. Master of Science (Research) dissertation. School of Health and Biomedical Sciences, College of Science, Engineering and Health, RMIT University

Stubbe DE (2020) Practicing cultural competence and cultural humility in the care of diverse patients. Focus 18(1):49–51

Tervalon M, Murray-Garcia J (1998) Cultural humility versus cultural competence: a critical distinction in defining physician training outcomes in multicultural education. J Health Care Poor Underserved 9(2):117–125

Truth and Reconciliation Commission of Canada. (2015). *Final Report of the Truth and Reconciliation Commission of Canada, Volume One: Summary: Honouring the Truth, Reconciling for the Future*. James Lorimer & Company

Ungunmerr MR (2017) To be listened to in her teaching: Dadirri: Inner deep listening and quiet still awareness. EarthSong J: Perspect Ecol Spirit Edu 3(4):14–15

United Nations (2007) Declaration on the Rights of Indigenous Peoples (UNDRIP). Available at: http://www.un.org/esa/socdev/unpfii/documents/DRIPS_en.pdf

Vindigni D (2004) Promoting the musculoskeletal Health of Indigenous Australians Living in Rural Communities. Aboriginal Health in Aboriginal communities. Doctoral thesis

Vindigni D, Polus B, Edgecombe G, Howard M, van Rotterdam J, Redpath F, Ellen E (2009) The STTEP: a model for musculoskeletal health care in marginalized communities. J Altern Complement Med 15(8):885–890

Vindigni D, Polus B, van Rotterdam J, da Costa C, Edgecombe G, Walsh M, Howard M, Bromwell T, Biasbas A, Cohen M, Patterson C (2011) The sustainable training, treatment, employment program model: effects of manual therapy on musculoskeletal pain and limitation in a Filipino squatter community. J Manip Physiol Ther 34(6):381–387

Williams R (1999) Cultural safety—what does it mean for our work practice? Aust N Z J Public Health 23(2):213–214

World Health Organization (WHO) (2017) Health is a fundamental human right. Available at: https://www.who.int/news-room/commentaries/detail/health-is-a-fundamental-human-right

Yeager KA, Bauer-Wu S (2013) Cultural humility: essential foundation for clinical researchers. Appl Nurs Res 26(4):251–256

Chapter 13
A Holistic Ecosystem of Health and Healthcare: Spirit, Mind and Body

Sandra Jones and Dein Vindigni OAM

Abstract The aim of this chapter is to discuss the inclusion of spirituality as part of the holistic ecosystem of health and healthcare. This is explored through the lens of the Ancient Indigenous Wisdoms of the Australian First Nations People. First, a reflection on the relationship between the 3P agencies of health and healthcare and the 6Ls of Ancient Indigenous Wisdoms is undertaken (see Chaps. 11 and 12). A second reflection is undertaken of the relationship between the 6Ls of Ancient Indigenous Wisdoms and the modes of cognition, methods of action and tenets of lead(er)ship identified in the ecologies assembled to explain the implications of the adoption of a Complexity science lens (see Chaps. 8, 9, 10). The conclusion reached is that, before a truly inclusive holistic ecosystem of health and healthcare can be imagined, there is need to add the spiritual to the mind-body focus of mainstream Western approaches to health and healthcare.

13.1 Complexity in Context

We have discussed in earlier chapters that Complexity science recognizes the importance of context in which things behave according to their nature. Boulton, Allen, and Bowman (2015, p. 54) described this in the words "what we are is contingent on the context in which we find conjoining … We … are emergent patterns and may

S. Jones (✉)
Business and Law College, RMIT University, Melbourne, VIC, Australia

D. Vindigni OAM
STEM College, RMIT University, Melbourne, VIC, Australia
e-mail: dein.vindigni@rmit.edu.au

S. Jones, D. Vindigni OAM (eds.), *Health and Healthcare in Complexity*,
https://doi.org/10.1007/978-981-96-0515-6_13

shift into new patterns." This, they claimed, creates a tension between formal patterns of stability and changing aspects of phenomena that creates emergent patterns. They described this as similar to pre-Socratic thinking in which "there is a sense of the world as changing whilst nevertheless manifesting coherence and patterning....a sense of flow and interconnections and impermanence" (Boulton et al. 2015, p. 53). This thinking is very similar to ideas, emerging in the East, in Hinduism and Buddhism, and in China in Daoism, that challenge unambiguous cause and effect relationships and instead adopt a more holistic philosophy focused on interconnections between constituent elements, including spirituality (Boulton et al. 2015). The inclusion of spirituality requires extension of the holistic biopsychological 'lived' body approach of Complexity science (see Chap. 2). That is, while Complexity science recognizes interconnections and co-creation that are interdependent and mutually determining, influenced by episodic change rather than incremental and continuous change, it is comparatively silent on issues of spirituality. If, as is claimed, there is need to focus on the particularity of events, there is need for spirituality to be acknowledged "'the devil is in the detail'...knowing the 'minute particulars' is necessary to understanding what emerges" (Boulton et al. 2015, p. 55). This is highlighted in the words of an Australian Indigenous Elder:

'we are one with the world (Kakkib li'Dthia Warrawee'a 2002).

13.2 A Holistic Ecosystem of Health and Healthcare: Spirit, Mind and Body

Reflection on the potential of a holistic ecosystem of health and healthcare to acknowledge, and include, the spiritual as a third element of the mind-body focus of mainstream Western approaches to health and healthcare was undertaken by the authors using the lens of the Ancient Indigenous Wisdoms of Australian Indigenous People (see Chaps. 11 and 12).

First, reflection was undertaken of the relationship between the 3P agencies of health and healthcare: Principles and Purposes (P1); People in Place (P2); and Practices and Processes (P3) and the 6Ls of (the Australian Aboriginal) Ancient Indigenous Wisdoms, Lore (L1); Love (L2); Look (L3); Listen (L4); Learn (L5); and Lead or Leave Alone (L6).[1] This resulted in identification of a potential relationship (summarized in the two inner circles of Fig. 13.1) between:

1. Principles and Purposes (P1) and the 2 Ls of Lore and Love (based on a potential understanding of the human-nature-spiritual connection).
2. People in Place (P2) and the 3Ls of; Learn (grounded in sharing varied perspectives), Love (for Community) and Lore (based in cultural humility and patience).

[1] See Chaps. 11 and 12.

3. Practice and Process (P3) and the 3Ls of; Look and Listen (grounded in notions of truth and honor), Lead (based in relationships), and Leave Alone (to explore emergent futures).

Second, reflection was undertaken of the relationship between the 6Ls and the modes of cognition, methods of action and tenets of lead(er)ship identified in the ecologies presented in Chaps. 8, 9, and 10. The findings are set out below (summarized in the middle and outer circles of Fig. 13.1). This resulted in identification of a potential relationship between:

1. Lore, systems thinking and sensemaking.
2. Love (*human-nature interconnection*) and social ecological thinking.
3. Love (*individual and spiritual connection*) and reflective thinking.
4. Learn (*varied perspectives*) and distributive engagement.
5. Love (*for Community*) and networking.
6. Lore (*cultural humility and patience*) and participatory action research.
7. Look and Listen (*from humility for truth*) and reflexive practice (to observe patterns).
8. Lead (*based in relationships*) and the tenets of leadership (to co-create the future).
9. Leave Alone (*waiting for emergent futures*) and emergent patterns.

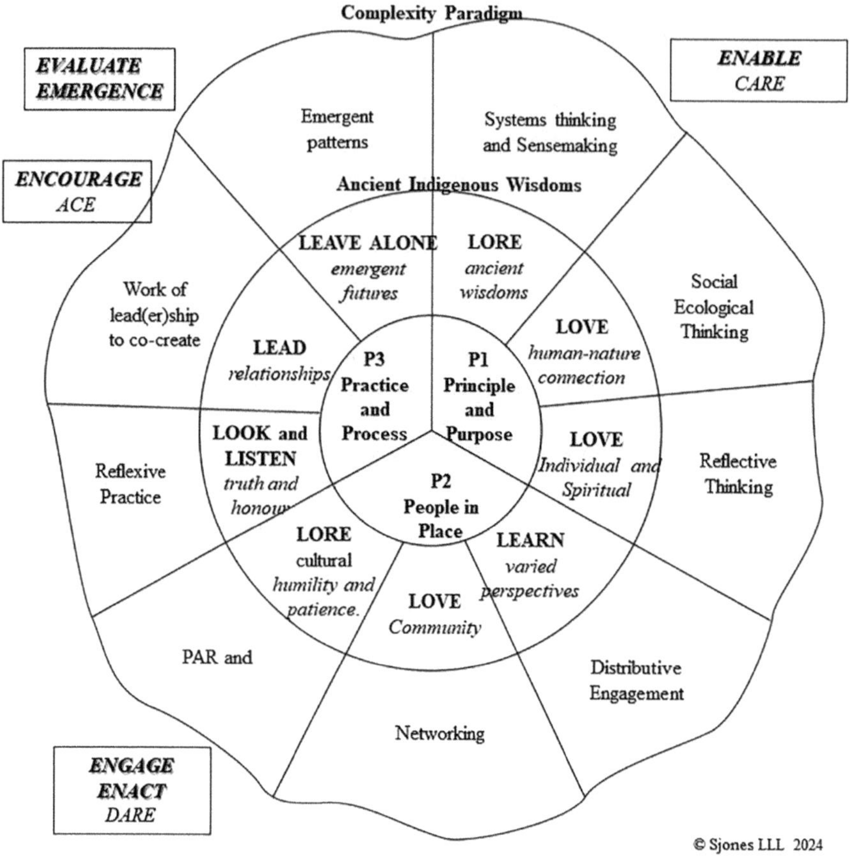

Fig. 13.1 A Holistic Spiritual Inclusive Ecosystem (HSIE): Conjoining Western and Indigenous Approaches to Health and Healthcare

Third, based on the proposed Holistic Spirital Inclusive Ecosystem (HSIE) of Health and Healthcare (Fig. 13.1), reflection was undertaken with the aim of creating a resource to assist individuals and groups to identify opportunities to include the spiritual in a holistic ecosystem of health and healthcare. The reflection took into account the descriptor of the 6Ls of the Ancient Indigenous Wisdoms. It resulted in the design of a resource with 15 reflection prompts. termed the *Self Enabling Ecology for Reflection on Spirituality (Template 13.1 SEER S).*

Template 13.1 Self-Enabling Ecology of Reflection on Spirit (SEER S)

Use the reflection prompts to identify examples of the conjoining of Western (3P agencies) and Indigenous approach to the spirit underpinning…

3P agencies of health and healthcare	LORE (1)	*Ancient* LOVE (2)	*Indigenous* LOOK (3)	*Wisdoms* LISTEN (4)	LEARN (5)	LEAD (OR LEAVE ALONE (L6)
Principles and purposes (P1) *…encourage understanding of the organisation as a whole*	*…Ancient knowledge as wisdoms required to live in harmony with all creation*	*…respect for Indigenous spiritual and cultural practices*	*…awaken perceptive capacities to notice and observe Earth-Kin*	*…share the gifts of creation*	*…contentment comes from finding meaning and purpose through learning and growth*	*…achieve the best outcome for all through establishing relationships with people and Country*
People in place (P2) *…enable collaborative, reciprocal relationships*		*…relationships built in good intentions and motivations*	***…**people actively watch and observe nature (bush)*	*…gain knowledge by looking and listening*	*…engage in community through learn through cultural respect and community*	*…engage humans in balance with nature*
Practices and processes (P3) ***…**encourage interdependent systems to clarify meaning and springboard collaborative action*	*…Ancient knowledge as wisdoms required to live in harmony with each other*	*…encourage exchange of stories*	*…observe and begin to appreciate acceptable (and unacceptable) practices*	*…listen with humility respect and patience to individual stories*	*…look and listen to gain understanding of local culture knowledge*	*…design teaching and learning that is locally oriented, & designed to restore ecological balance*

13.3 Conclusion

This chapter explored the potential of adapting the proposed holistic ecosystem of health and healthcare based in the principles of Complexity to include the element of the spiritual (to add to the current Western mind-body focus.) While reflections revealed some potential, they also highlight the need for research before change of this order can be achieved.

References

Boulton JG, Allen PM, Bowman C (2015) Embracing complexity: strategic perspectives for an Age of Turbulence. Oxford University Press

Kakkib li'Dthia Warrawee'a (2002) There once was a tree called Deru / Kakkib li'Dthia Warrawee'a, Thorsons Pymble, NSW

Part III
Paradigm Shift for Health and Healthcare: From the edge

Part III of this book seeks to explore the factors that contribute to a successful paradigm shift to more collaborative a holistic ecosystem of health and healthcare. This is achieved through reflection on five projects that were each designed to use a collaborative partnership to provide integrated health and healthcare to people living with disadvantage. Although these projects were not guided by the ecologies assembled in Prt II, the editors applied a reflection-on-practice approach. Four reflective techniques were employed: Narrative, Concept Mapping and Critical Incident were used to analyze the project experiences of the 3P agencies of health and heathcare and Appreciative Inquiry to identify the challenges for collaboration in seeking to replace the habitual practice in health and healthcare. Given the finding in Chap. 10 of the contribution of the 6Es of Distributed Leadership to collaboration, the Appreciative Inquiry adopted the 6Es to report the findings. While it is acknowledged that these projects preceded the ecologies identified in Chaps. 8, 9 and 10, the findings do highlight how a project-based approach ('from the edge') may contribute to a successful paradigm change in health and healthcare.

Chapter 14
Paradigm Shift for Health and Healthcare: Reflection-on-Practice

Sandra Jones

Abstract The aim of this chapter is to explore how application of reflective practice can be used to identify future change to assist a paradigm shift to a holistic ecosystem for health and healthcare. It explains how reflection-on-practice can be used to identify lessons learnt from projects that were designed as collaborative partnerships to provide integrated health and healthcare to people living with disadvantage. Four reflective techniques are described: Narrative, Concept Mapping, Critical Incident Analysis, and Appreciative Inquiry. The techniques are tailored to the purpose of this book, first, to analyze the project experience for each of the 3P agencies of health and healthcare: Principles and Purpose (P1); People in Place (P2); and Practices and Processes (P3). Second, to undertake critical reflection of the projects to identify the challenges for collaboration in seeking to replace the habitual practice in health and healthcare of hierarchies of decision making.

14.1 Introduction

Change of the magnitude proposed by a paradigm shift to a holistic ecosystem of health and healthcare is challenging. This explains the limited degree of meaningful change that has occurred due to the ongoing influence of Cartesian science; innate resistance to change and the desire by many to retain existing structures of power and influence. As authors, we accept the challenges of finding ways to help people to reflect on mindsets and overarching worldviews, and to critique some long-term beliefs, to consider what is needed to achieve a change in paradigms (Boulton et al. 2015). We accept that the challenges require more than simply a map or toolkit of actions to implement meaningful change. Given these challenges, we

S. Jones (✉)
Business and Law College, RMIT University, Melbourne, VIC, Australia

S. Jones, D. Vindigni OAM (eds.), *Health and Healthcare in Complexity*,
https://doi.org/10.1007/978-981-96-0515-6_14

maintain that change is more likely to come from the 'edge' rather than from those entrenched in the current paradigm. This chapter discusses how reflection-on-practice can be used to identify lessons learnt from projects implemented from 'the edge'. The projects chosen were each designed as collaborative partnerships aimed to provide integrated health and healthcare services for people living with disadvantage. Four reflective practice techniques are chosen. Three reflective techniques: narrative, concept mapping and critical incident analysis; first are used to explore the contributions of the 3P agencies of health and healthcare: Principles and Purpose (P1); People in Place (P2) and Practices and Processes (P3) with the intention of producing knowledge about application in practice. The fourth, appreciative inquiry, is applied as a critical reflection lens to focus on change from the bottom-up identifying the challenges for collaboration in seeking to replace the habitual practice in health and healthcare of hierarchies of decision-making. Given the relationship between the 6Es and collaboration identified in Chap. 10, the appreciative inquiry adopts the 6Es (see Chap. 10) Engage; Enable; Enact; Encourage; Evaluate and Emerge.

14.2 Why Reflective Practice

14.2.1 Philosophy of Reflective Practice

Reflective inquiry, or reflective practice, is part of the epistemology of practice that Schön (1983, 1987) discussed as designed to extend technical problem-solving to acknowledge a broad context. Reflection has been described by Boud et al. (1998, p. 19) as "a generic term for those intellectual and affective activities in which individuals engage to explore their experiences in order to lead to new understandings and appreciation." Reflective thinking is described as a "a process of thinking, feeling, imagining and learning by considering what has happened in the past, what might be happening if things had been done differently, what is currently happening and what could possibly happen in the future" (Rolfe 2011, p. 13). Applied to higher education, Harvey et al. (2016, p. 9) described reflective practice as "a deliberate and conscientious approach that employs a person's cognitive, emotional and somatic capacities to mindfully contemplate on past, present or future (intended or planned) actions in order to learn, better understand and potentially improve future actions." Applied to healthcare, Ghaye and Lillyman (2010, pp. 167–168) described reflective practice as involving "a combination of a disposition towards our work (a frame of mind or mind-set) together with understanding, embracing and utilizing a set of principles and skills… to provide the opportunity for us to become even better at what we do." Johns (1995, p. 25) claimed that when applied to nursing, reflection is simply "the method to access, make sense of, and learn through experience."

14.2.2 Purpose of Reflective Practice

The purpose of reflective practice is not to simply tell a story but to provide a means to make sense of the narrative. This involves considering how to replicate and amplify success, to help individuals and groups to frame and reframe experiences into new options and alternatives, to understand the link and interdependence between human and organizational agency, to contribute to lifelong learning in workplaces, and to explore changes to individual and collective practice to improve quality.

14.2.3 Contribution of Reflective Practice

Schön (1983, 1987) described the outcome of reflection as helping to resolve uncertainties or 'confusing messes' by enabling people to gain personal insight from practice experience to inform decision-making. Applying this to quality improvement in healthcare, Ling et al. (2008, p. 2) claimed that reflection enables practitioners to step back from the immediate challenge of delivering care to "reflect on the benefits of alternate ways of delivering care and, where appropriate, challenging how care is delivered."

Reflective practice complements evidence-based practice (EBP) that is the dominant approach to research in healthcare (Sackett et al. 1996). Underpinning EBP is a strong research culture with a framework that enables service planning, decision-making, and sustained integration of evidence-based healthcare (Misso et al. 2016; Rolfe 2011; Farmer and Weston 2002). Kane and Trochim (2009) claimed that reflective practice contributes an integrated approach through which social research adds value to evidence-based practice. Critical reflective practice adds a further dimension by which practice is examined for its implications. Jasper and Rolfe (2011, p. 5) explained that "critical reflection goes beyond the simple recollection and description of events and involves some kind of analysis of the meaning and implications of what we are reflecting on." The underlying assumption is that reflective practice leads to change in practice. Jasper and Rolfe (2011, p. 6) claimed that "if reflective practice is not translated back into practice it is of little use and is ultimately nothing more than an empty intellectual exercise." Finally, reflective practice can encourage collaboration and participation by:

> [enabling] co-researchers with different perspectives and ways of understanding, as well as iterative cycles of action and research, *[to]* provide a robust model to increase our understanding of complex situations, while designing and monitoring interventions. (Hughes 2008, p. 390)

Reflective practice in healthcare has been used to both assist individuals to grow through a process of self-appraisal (Carr and Kemmis 1986) and to serve the collective interest of teams. It helps to link personal and professional values with practice, healthcare intentions with action, and individuals with team development. This is important in a clinical context "which oscillates at the boundary between stability and chaos" (Ghaye and Lillyman 2010, p. 100). Reflective practice in Indigenous health and healthcare is assumed to take part within the practice of incorporating the interconnected state of spiritual, communal, and ecosystem equilibrium and well-being (Nettleton et al. 2007)

14.2.4 *Forms of Reflective Practice*

Schön (1983, 1987) differentiated between three forms of practical knowledge: 'knowing-in-action,' 'reflection-in-practice,' and 'reflection-on-practice'. Each enables the reframing of problems to assist understanding of complexity and contributing to improving practice:

- Knowing-in-action is discussed in a previous chapter[1] under the term reflexivity, as one of the methods of action that contribute to the assemblage of an ecology of actions to build relationships.
- Reflection-in-practice occurs when doing and thinking occur simultaneously to influence decisions being made. This differs from problem-solving as it leads to a change in the practitioner's view (of self, values, and beliefs). This was discussed under the term reflective thinking,[2] as one of the modes of thinking that contribute to the assemblage of an ecology of cognition.
- Reflection-on-practice occurs in retrospect by enabling a "stepping back and checking out what we thought and said earlier" (Ghaye and Lillyman 2010, p. 98). Greenwood (1993, p. 1185) referred to reflection-on-practice as providing the opportunity for a 'cognitive postmortem,' after the situation has occurred, during which the practitioner looks back on the experiences to explore again the understanding brought to them in light of the outcome. This is applied in the following chapters to enable a postmortem of the experiences of five projects designed to provide integrated health and healthcare services through collaborative partnerships.

14.3 Processes and Techniques of Reflective Practice

Kim (1999) identified three phases of reflective practice:

(i) A descriptive phase in which narrative is used to describe events, processes, or practice (actions, thoughts, and feelings) which are then examined for their genuineness or comprehensiveness.

---

[1] See Chap. 9.

[2] See Chap. 8.

(ii) A reflective phase during which narrative is analyzed against espoused theories (scientific, ethical, and esthetic), situations, and intentions and then combined with self-awareness to produce knowledge about application in practice. The focus is on observing the emergence of new patterns or the disturbance of old patterns.

(iii) A critical reflective phase[3] that may include challenges to the status quo or routine and habitual practice. It may focus on identifying conflicts, distortions, or inconsistencies alongside perceived emancipatory or change processes. This may occur through a mix of learning and change in practice as well as through self-critique and emancipation (Ghaye and Lillyman 2010). The primary source of data is "our own experiences…data is generated and collated through the rigorous application of one or more systematic reflective frameworks, which constitute our data collection methods" (Jasper and Rolfe 2011, p. 6).

We have chosen four reflective techniques: Narrative combined with Critical Incident Analysis and Concept Mapping to observe the emergence of new patterns and describe the disturbance of old patterns. This is identified through a focus on the 3P agencies of health and healthcare. Appreciative Inquiry, also is used to identify challenges to the status quo, using the 6Es (see Chap. 10), to identify the challenge of collaboration for the habitual practice in health and healthcare of hierarchies in decision-making.

14.3.1 Narrative

Narrative is used during the descriptive phase to present a story:

> where a teller, motivated by unexpected events, describes to a recipient of the story a sequence of purposeful actions with a plot (a beginning, middle, and end) set in a particular context and arranged according to a temporal structure. It is the inter-subjective nature of the dialogue in encounters between patients and health care practitioners and among practitioners that constitutes a fundamentally communicative act—a narrative. (Engel et al. 2008, pp. 6–7)

Gray (2009, p. 267) stated that "Storytelling has been a way to communicate information, learn about life, transmit culture, make sense of experience, and express one's emotions since primitive forms of language emerged ages ago." Narrative has long been used in healthcare to turn a private experience into a valuable public learning experience, particularly with patents and as a key communication strategy. Gray (2009, p. 259) explained:

> Within medical training, students must learn both the art and science of medicine, there are issues of learning both the art and science of medicine, understanding the basic science of disease as well as the individual patient's illness experience and its influence on health. Narrative is a key communication strategy and concept crucial in all of these interrelated

[3] Habermas (1987) went further to label this an emancipatory phase.

> issues, as human beings are all storytellers. Understanding patients' experiences in the clinical encounter and in clinical training through their stories, and communicating health information in a persuasive, easily understood manner in various settings may be accomplished through the use of narrative, as a clinical counselling strategy, an information-gathering technique, and a teaching tool.

Engel et al. (2008) combined their expertise from social science, clinical practice, and counselling, to explore the opportunity provided by reflective practice to conceptualize a narrative of healthcare practices within a new framework of shared disciplines. Through their experience, they highlighted the opportunity to apply their shared reflection to develop skills required to engage in relationship-centered care and patient-centered care. Charon (2008, p. x) explained that such cross-discipline reflection requires a more diverse range of skills beyond clinical skills to include "reading and telling complex stories, reasoning with stories, writing reflectively, compassionate presence, mindful listening, practicing empathy, and exercising the moral imagination and linguistics." Gray (2009, p. 267) explained that lived experiences attempt to make sense of actions, motives, and consequences, as well as interactions, relationships, and emotions:

> When narratives are internally formulated, verbalised, or written down, human beings are making sense of and recreating experiences and essentially weaving these experiences into their lives and communicating these experiences to others.

14.3.2 Critical Incident Analysis

Critical incident analysis generally occurs during the descriptive phase to reflect upon important (significant) issues that arise in a systematic manner. A critical incident is a retrospective event that generates an action, which, due to its retrospective perspective, can only be determined as critical after the event. The incident is deemed to be critical when the subsequent action is sufficient in itself to allow conclusions and predictions to be made by the person carrying out the act. In complexity thinking there is an emphasis on the importance of being sensitive to critical junctures which may become the moments for radical change to emerge (Boulton et al. 2015). Fridlund et al. (2017) identified a critical incident as follows:

1. An event with a distinct beginning and a distinct end, with the resultant actions' intent as well as its effect needing to be clear with a tangible outcome.
2. Involving an 'extra something' that distinguishes it from the common or everyday incident that the participant does not remember in the same way.
3. Triggering an action which has a significant impact on the final result.
4. Possibly consisting of more than one significant incident.

14.3.3 Concept Mapping

Concept mapping occurs during the reflective phase to identify key ideas and concepts that act as a catalyst for change. It involves a mixed methods approach that can be used to structure conceptualization to address complex issues in health and healthcare and to provide a framework that can guide action planning, program development, or evaluation and measurement. Van Bon-Martens et al. (2017) state the advantages of concept mapping are as follows:

1. Integration of tacit knowledge from different groups of stakeholders including practitioners, patients, other professionals, citizens, and managers.
2. Engagement of decision-makers from the public health community.
3. Crossing of disciplinary boundaries and the combination of quantitative and qualitative research methods.
4. Theoretical development that can occur as the ideas of different groups, using a variety of visual means, make inferences possible about the relations between those ideas.

14.3.4 Critical Reflection: Appreciative Inquiry

Appreciative inquiry generally occurs during critical reflection phase designed to provide the opportunity to move away from a traditional deficit problem-solving approach to a strengths-based approach. This is achieved by inviting a focus on the positive dynamics of relationships between people through strengthening "our collective capacity to imagine and build a better future" (Cooperrider 2001, p. 34), by focusing on appreciation, affirmation, and being open to positive dialog about future possibilities (Cooperrider 1986). Building from Reed (2007), Trajkovski et al. (2013, p. 95) stated that in adopting a participatory approach, appreciative inquiry offers a flexible framework to facilitate change from the grass roots up. It lends itself to building effective partnerships and collaborations that can be used to meet specific needs of an organization.

Ghaye and Lillyman (2010) identified four forms of appreciative intent: knowing (being selectively attentive to the positive and essential), relating (valuing and affirming the worth of others through interactions), actioning (inspiring action by positive intent, ethic of care, and organizational structures and processes that empower all involved to reach their highest potential), and organizing (committing to building trust among multidisciplinary teams, getting ideas to improve practice from everywhere, readiness for innovation, becoming emotionally intelligent, and developing learning-enriched clinical areas). Cooperrider et al. (2008) identified a four-part iterative process: (i) discovering (appreciate what is working well), (ii) dreaming (envisage what might be or what needs to be changed), (iii) designing (What are we learning or what should we be learning?), and iv) further designing (Where do we go from here? How do we empower, learn, and adjust/improvise for sustainability?). We use appreciative inquiry based in the reflections of agents who facilitated change in projects coupled with analysis by an external expert on complexity and leadership.

14.4 Discussion

The projects chosen for the reflection-on-practice have several common, and some unique, characteristics that make them suitable for our purpose:

1. Each project was designed to improve the health and healthcare of a particular group of people living with disadvantage (economic, age, culture). This enabled consideration of issues of access and equity discussed in Chap. 6 and consideration of a patient-centered focus discussed in Chap. 5.
2. Each project involved collaboration primarily between healthcare professionals from allied and complementary medicine but also medical professionals. This enabled consideration of issues related to integration of the professions discussed in Chap. 4.
3. Each project was underpinned by a collaborative partnership formed between not-for-profit provider(s), a university, and various philanthropic funding bodies. This enabled consideration of collaborative partnerships and leadership discussed in Chap. 7.
4. One project was underpinned by a collaborative partnership designed to train local Indigenous health providers in complementary medicine as discussed in Chap. 13.
5. Each project has resulted in embedded and sustained outcomes.

Without prejudicing the findings from reflections on each project several common factors are identified as follows:

1. The importance of identifying, and agreeing on (formally or informally), Principles and Purpose (P1). This includes identification of a clear framework upon which roles, responsibilities and decision-making processes for collaboration is agreed. Despite the time this may take, the value in preventing misunderstanding during the project is emphasised.
2. The significance of ensuring that all relevant experts are involved, that diverse contexts and cultures are understood, and that engagement in decision making is shared, that is People in Place (P2).
3. The significance of agreement on a detailed plan of action that includes description of Processes and Practices (P3) to support and evaluate collaboration.

14.5 Conclusion

This chapter has highlighted the importance of reflection-on-practice to identify actions needed to support change from 'the edge' to encourage a paradigm change to a holistic ecosystem of health and healthcare. Four techniques of reflective practice are discussed and applied to five projects that had as their aim to establish a collaborative partnership to provide integrated health and healthcare to people living with disadvantage.

While these projects were undertaken before the ecologies assembled and the SEERs identified to assist change in Chap. 8, 9 and 10, the findings from the lessons learnt suggest that application of these ecologies and SEERs could assist future planning and sustainability of the change implemented. While these projects were primarily focused in the provision of allied and complementary health they did, overtime, include medical professionals. While each project was located within the domains of public and social healthcare, the findings are equally applicable to all healthcare. While each project aimed to establish a collaborative partnership, they were all challenged by how to differentiate between the project objective, and the aim of establishing a collaborative partnership. This resulted in each having difficulty in identifying the factors required for successful collaborative partnerships. The use of critical reflection assisted in addressing this challenge and helped identify the importance of obtaining agreement (formally and informally) on the Principles and Purposes (P1), engaging People in Place (P2), and designing Practices and Processes (P3) to support collaboration as well as to achieve the specific (health) purpose of the project.

References

Boud D, Keogh R, Walker D (1998) Promoting reflection in learning: a model. In: Boud D, Keogh R, Walker D (eds) Reflection: turning experiences into learning. Kogan Page, London

Boulton JG, Allen PM, Bowman C (2015) Embracing complexity: strategic perspectives for an Age of Turbulence. Oxford University Press

Nettleton C. et al. (2007) Utz Wachil: Findings from an International Study of Indigenous Perspectives on Health and Environment. EcoHealth 4:461–471. https://doi.org/10.1007/s10393-007-0138-9

Carr W, Kemmis S (1986) Becoming critical: education, knowledge and action research. Falmer Press, London

Charon R (2008) Narrative medicine: honoring the stories of illness. Oxford University Press

Cooperrider DL (1986) Appreciative inquiry: toward a methodology for understanding and enhancing organizational innovation. Western Reserve University, Cleveland, OH

Cooperrider D. (2001) Working Paper: appreciative inquiry: releasing the power of the positive question. Case western reserve university cleveland, oh united states. Available online at: http://appreciativeinquiry.case.edu/uploads/working_paper_Aand_power_positive_question.pd

Cooperrider DL, Whitney D, Stavros JM (2008) Appreciative inquiry handbook: for leaders of change, 2nd edn. Brunswick, OH, Crown Custom

Engel JD et al (2008) Narrative in Helath Care: Healing Patient, Practitionrs, Profession and Community. CRC Press: London. https://doi.org/10.1201/97813153833095
Farmer E, Weston K (2002) A conceptual model for capacity building in Australian primary health care research. Aust Fam Physician 31(12):1139–1142
Fridlund B, Henricson M, Mårtensson J (2017) Critical incident technique applied in nursing and healthcare sciences. SOJ Nursing Health Care 3(1):1–5. https://doi.org/10.15226/2471-6529/3/1/00125
Ghaye T, Lillyman S (2010) Reflection: principles and practices for healthcare professionals. Andrews UK Ltd.
Gray JB (2009) The power of storytelling: using narrative in the healthcare context. J Commun Healthc 2(3):258–273. https://doi.org/10.1179/cih.2009.2.3.258
Greenwood J (1993) Reflective practice: a critique of the work of Argyris and Schön. J Adv Nurs 18:1183–1187
Habermas (1987) Knowledge and human interest. Policy Press, Cambridge
Harvey M, Coulson D, McMaugh A (2016) Towards a theory of the ecology of reflection: Reflective practice for experiential learning in higher education. Journal of University Teaching and Learning Practice 13(2)
Hughes I (2008) Action Research in Health and Healthcare. Ch 25:381-393. In Reason P, Bradbury H (Eds.) Sage handbook of action research. SAGE pubs. London
Jasper M, Rolfe G (2011). Critical reflection and the emergence of professional knowledge, Ch. 1:1-8. In Rolfe G, Jasper M, Freshwater D (eds) Critical Reflections in Practice: Generating Knowledge for Care. 2nd Edition. Springer Nature Ltd Red Globe Press
Johns C (1995) The value of reflective practice for nursing. J Clin Nurs 4:23–30
Kane M, Trochim W.M (2009) Concept mapping for applied social research. In: The Sage handbook of applied social research methods, pp. 435–474. SAGE Publications, Inc., Thousand Oaks
Kim HS (1999) Critical reflective inquiry for knowledge development in nursing practice. Journal of advanced nursing 29(5):1205–1212.
Ling T, Soper B, Buxton M et al (2008) An evaluation of the health foundation's engaging with quality initiative. The Health Foundation, London
Misso ML, Ilic D, Haines TP et al (2016) Development, implementation and evaluation of a clinical research engagement and leadership capacity building program in a large Australian health care service. BMC Med Educ 16:13. https://doi.org/10.1186/s12909-016-0525-421. BMC Open access
Reed J (2007) Appreciative inquiry: research for change. Sage, Thousand Oaks, CA
Rolfe G (2011) Knowledge and practice, Ch.2. In: Rolfe J, Jasper M, Freshwater D (eds) Critical reflection in practice, 2nd edn. Palgrave Macmillan, Basingstoke, Hampshire, pp 11–29
Sackett DL, Rosenberg W, McGray JA et al (1996) Evidence based medicine: what it is and what it isn't. BMJ 312:71–72. https://doi.org/10.1136/bmj.312.7023.7
Schön D (1983) The reflective practitioner: how professionals think in action. Basic Books, New York
Schön D (1987) Educating the reflective practitioner. San Francisco, Jossey Base
Trajkovski S, Schmied V, Vickers M et al (2013) Using appreciative inquiry to transform. Contemp Nurse 45(1):95–100
Trochim W, Kane M (2005) Concept mapping: an introduction to structured conceptualization in health care. Int J Qual Health Care 17(3):187–191
van Bon-Martens Marja JH, van de Goorb Ien AM, van Oers Hans AM (2017) Concept mapping as a method to enhance evidence-based public health. Eval Program Plann 60:213–228

Chapter 15
Applying Reflection-on-Practice to a Collaborative Health Partnership for the Disadvantaged: The 'Bone Men' Project

Dein Vindigni OAM, Barbara Polus, and Sandra Jones

Abstract This chapter presents the findings from applying reflection-on-practice to a health project that was instigated in 1989 as a collaborative partnership. First, a descriptive narrative is combined with concept mapping and critical incident analysis, to explore the project experience of each of the 3P agencies of health and healthcare. Second, a critical reflection is undertaken, using appreciative inquiry, to identify challenges for collaboration in seeking to replace the habitual practice in health and healthcare of hierarchies of decision making.

15.1 Introduction

The project presented in this chapter was initiated in 1989 as a collaborative partnership between an allied and complementary health professional (a chiropractor—henceforth termed Agent A1) and the CEO of a not-for-profit (NFP) Mission. The project is termed the 'Bone Men' in recognition of the terminology used by patients. The NFP Mission was initially established to assist people resident in the immediate local community who were experiencing homelessness or disadvantage (Vindigni 1990). After 2 years of operation, a university that offered a degree program in chiropractic was added as a third partner in the collaborative partnership.

The reflection-on-practice in this chapter is undertaken by two of the agents: the health professional (chiropractor) who initiated the project (A1) and the academic who championed the collaboration with the university [A2]). First, a descriptive narrative is combined with concept mapping and critical incident analysis

D. Vindigni OAM (✉) · B. Polus
STEM College, RMIT University, Melbourne, VIC, Australia
e-mail: dein.vindigni@rmit.edu.au

S. Jones
Business and Law College, RMIT University, Melbourne, VIC, Australia

S. Jones, D. Vindigni OAM (eds.), *Health and Healthcare in Complexity*,
https://doi.org/10.1007/978-981-96-0515-6_15

to analyse the experience for each of the 3P agencies of health and healthcare. This is reported in Sect. 15.2 and Sect. 15.3. Second, critical reflection is undertaken using appreciative inquiry to identify the challenges for collaboration in seeking to replace the habitual practice of hierarchies of decision making in health and healthcare. This is reported in Sect. 15.4. This stage engaged an expert in Complexity science and leadership to assist a focus on further design (where do we go from here) an how to empower, learn and adjust/improvise for sustainability.

15.2 Narrative, Concept Mapping and Critical Incident Analysis

15.2.1 Principle and Purpose (P1)

In June 1989, a haggard and stooped man, laying aside his trepidation and mistrust, shuffled through the doors of an inner-city not-for-profit Mission (hereafter termed the Mission). He had heard a rumour on the streets that there were people there with a special touch, and so he had come in search of the 'Bone Men'. Though he had come voluntarily, upon his first meeting with one of these 'Bone Men', he still asked suspiciously, "You're not gonna crack me, are ya?". (Agent A1)

Agent A1 reflects:

*The initial design of the project was informed by my experience and knowledge of similar charity-based voluntary health clinics in Calcutta, India and the USA. In 1989, I approached the CEO of a Not-for-Profit Mission in Victoria (Australia) about the possibility of establishing a voluntary health clinic to provide free-for-service Medical, Allied Health and Complementary health services to residents in the local community who were living with disadvantage. My proposal was influenced by the, then recent, finding of an Australian Government Report that had identified the importance of integrating chiropractic across the community, especially for people experiencing socio-economic disadvantage (*Layton Report 1986*). At that time, chiropractic treatment was only available to individuals with private health insurance or to those who could afford to pay privately (*Marthick-Hone et al. 2022*). Further, many people living with disadvantage would shy away from chiropractic services either because they did not understand their function or they were considered to be something that only affluent people could afford. The CEO agreed to provide a space within the Mission grounds for the Clinic as its principle and purpose were in accord with the founding principle of the Mission "to assist people living in the local area who were experiencing homelessness or disadvantage, to find shelter, food, care and support."*

An (informal) agreement was reached for a Clinic to be established under a philosophy which recognised the importance of 'build(ing) a sense of self-worth – empowering people to respond to their intrinsic value and to take great control of their own lives'. This was seen as the first step towards achieving the goal of 'comprehensive health regardless of social or economic barriers'.

15.2.2 People in Place (P2)

The clinic represented a small but indispensable addition to the provision of vital services already provided by the Mission that included food, accommodation, and rehabilitation programs; additionally, it was a place of welcome and hospitality. The location of the Clinic within the physical domains of the Mission encouraged its use and contemporaneously discouraged the public from using the service, as most who entered the Mission were known to the Mission team and abided by the norms of conduct laid down by the team.

Agent A1 reflects:

The Clinic was initially staffed by volunteer chiropractors who shared a commitment to a holistic approach to the free provision of Allied healthcare for people living with disadvantage. Professionals from a variety of Allied and Complementary health fields, including podiatry, dermatology, occupational therapy, physiotherapy, dentistry, clinical psychology, massage therapy, naturopathy, optometry became engaged, as well as hairdressing that is not traditionally regarded as part of healthcare.

While chiropractors concern themselves primarily with restoring and maintaining the function of the spine, they also place emphasis on the importance of diet, exercise and lifestyle factors as indispensable concerns in promoting health ... correcting underlying foot conditions through podiatry often increases the likelihood of successfully treating problems of the spine ... removing the primary focus of irritations through orthotics followed by appropriate medical intervention, through dermatology, may assist skin disorders of the lower limbs, such as bunion formation due to poor footwear or skin ulceration secondary to diabetes ... natural remedies, through naturopathy, can play an important part in the health spectrum by augmenting the body's innate ability to help itself.

Those who frequented the Clinic brought a mix of backgrounds and life experiences with them. This resulted in many being reluctant to be treated, especially with the 'hands-on-healing' approach used by the clinicians.

Agent A1 reflects:

Some were born in the area, but a great many were displaced people from interstate or 'distant lands'. Some once held respected positions and enjoyed financial success but succumbed slowly to dependencies on alcohol and drugs. Many were alienated from their families. Others were single parents, homeless youth or sex workers. Some people suffered from mental illnesses and there were older persons who lived in the accommodation homes in the area.

Some barriers were broken after one of the patients termed us 'the Bone Men of St Kilda'. It also helped that the professional volunteers often spent time serving meals as well as providing clinical services. This led to strong relationships being built between the staff and attendees. The slow, but never tedious, mingling with the community acted as a valuable catalyst in pre-empting the many barriers to the integration of services. Over time, professionals recognised their role in not only assisting the physical needs but also the emotional and spiritual development of the individuals. As word spread, the waiting room of the Mission welcomed a steady stream of people from a variety of backgrounds waiting for treatment.

15.2.3 Practices and Processes (P3)

The one-room Clinic was initially established in the grounds of the Mission, but within 3 months, it had expanded to occupy three rooms.

Agent A1 reflects:

Resources and equipment were donated by private firms, individuals, practitioners and the university. The Clinic became a comfortable and safe place as volunteers welcomed each patient with cups of tea, cakes and biscuits. Most importantly, it was a place where they could come and chat.

The Clinic was mostly a happy, inviting place where staff, students and clients engaged on an equal footing and learned from each other. Many students commented that it was their best clinical experience.

As more students became engaged, the need to rent a building for the Clinic became evident. This required additional financing.

Agent A2 reflects:

I approached the Victorian Branch of a peak professional chiropractic body. They invited me to give a presentation to the Annual General Meeting and to request on-going support to pay rent and other expenses to maintain the Mission Clinic. My presentation was deliberately emotional and thought provoking. It was filled with photographs of the Mission and its community with the accompanying soundtrack of Neil Diamond's Jonathon Livingston Seagull. The presentation was successful, and they agreed to fund the Clinic (A3).

15.2.4 Evaluation

Evaluation of the effectiveness of the Clinic was undertaken using a mix of quantitative and qualitative measures.

Agent A1 reflects:

Formal qualitative measures included data on how many sessions and appointments were offered. By 1990, the health Clinic had operated over 90 sessions, averaging three hours each session and over 600 recorded appointments. Links had also been established with two other outreach programmes. Over time, the health Clinic expanded to include a drop-in centre. Anecdotal feedback from patients and practitioners was informally recorded. Mission workers and volunteers reported that many accommodation-home patients awaited their special hand massage with childlike anticipation. They also found that certain individuals receiving care for a low-back complaint or neck conditions began to pay more attention to personal hygiene and even to keenly adhere to suggestions for improving dietary habits.

As we were quick to learn, the people of the local area were remarkably honest in their observations of others. Just as signs of appreciation were made clearly visible with a job that was seen to be well done, we also learnt quickly if we had stepped out of line. There was no opportunity to hide behind stethoscopes or white coats in this setting. Practitioners soon realised the need to embrace the maxim of selecting the treatment which suited the client rather than forcing the client to conform to a pre-established treatment regime.

Since its initial establishment, the Clinic has expanded its role as a 'Wellness Place' designed to address the impacts of trauma, addiction, isolation, and chronic ill-health through a range of groups, educational programs, and complementary and allied health therapies.

15.3 Critical Incident Analysis

15.3.1 People in Place (P2): Addition of a University as a Partner

Within 2 years (in 1991), a large university which offered a degree in chiropractic was added as a third partner. A formal agreement was reached for students to participate in professional practice experience and to provide free care for people living with disadvantage.

Agent A2 reflects:

I was informed by a chiropractic student of the Open Day being held at the Mission Clinic. While in attendance, I thought about the possibilities for both chiropractic students and the Mission community of students providing musculoskeletal health care for people living with disadvantage. I reported back to my then Head of department (chiropractic) about the concept of a student chiropractic clinic. He initially seemed disinterested, and as I had competing demands on my time, no progress was made. Two years later, I was called back into the Head of Department's office. I was then informed that a student clinic could be set up at the Mission and I could lead the initiative if I was still interested.

While there was an initial (informal) agreement to collaborate between the CEO of the Mission and Agent A1, as the student Clinic, some confusion arose. This was due to the addition of a secondary purpose of providing professional practice opportunities for students (university focus), to that of providing free healthcare (Mission focus). This resulted in Agent A1 and A2 having to spend more time on building and maintaining relationships.

15.3.2 People in Place: Appointment of Clinic Coordinator

As the physical capacity of the Clinic expanded, so did the hours of opening, from the initial 2.5 days to 3 days a week. A Clinic Coordinator was appointed by the Mission to help establish and assist the operation of the Clinic. This was initially on a part-time basis, but it quickly increased to a full-time position as the Clinic Coordinator became indispensable to the operation of the Clinic.

Agent A1 reflects:

Those with experience in even a single-practitioner clinic will testify to the indispensable need for a sound organisational and administrative base without which even the most worthwhile project will falter. The Clinic Co-ordinator required not only a firm commitment to the Clinic's philosophy and a variety of organisational skills but a thorough understanding of the principles and workings of the Mission and the local Welfare Organisation which was affiliated with the Mission. The role of the Co-ordinator included liaising with the Mission workers and leaders as well as outside networks to ensure that they were all informed of developments and strategies and that they maintained a unity of purpose within the health team while balancing individual needs. This communication was fostered through regular newsletters, a comments book, informal discussions and (regular) meetings. The role also included structuring the clinical timetables and introducing new practitioners and visitors to the Clinic. Finally, there were general administration tasks associated with funding and resources.

15.3.3 Practices and Processes: Establishing Formal System and Meetings for Communication

Agent A1 reflects:

Mission staff were initially invited to a session in which the philosophy and practice of chiropractic were explained, and ideas for working as a team were exchanged. Following a visit to a local rooming home, a basic anatomy and therapeutic massage course (3x2 hour) was designed for Mission staff, to qualify them to provide face and hands massage. From this beginning, some Mission workers began to incorporate some of the techniques into regular accommodation home-visitations.

However, building relationships did not come without its challenges.

Agent A2 reflects:

An invitation was extended from the Mission to myself and students to have lunch in the Mission dining hall. During lunch, I asked an Indigenous woman sitting at the next table what her name was. For me, this was a way of starting a conversation. I immediately learned this was the wrong approach. She grabbed me by my hair and asked very sternly, "Who's asking?" A valuable lesson was learned.

To facilitate improved communication between all the disciplines, a system to generate smooth rosters and regulate appointments was introduced.

Agent A1 reflects:

Problems associated with the use of abbreviations and terminology are not unique to the Mission Health Programme; indeed they present a universal challenge to health workers. Nevertheless, we found this attempt at standardisation worthwhile. A colour-coded filing system was donated to the Mission for the use of all health workers. Each client's file was colour-coded, depending on predetermined criteria. For instance, every heath discipline was represented by a colour which was placed in a particular column. Colours in other columns might indicate the presenting complaint or may represent contra-indications of treatment or a recommendation to speak with staff prior to consultation. The colours and columns could be mixed and matched depending on the requirement. In this way, all client particulars were kept together, stored safely and were easily accessible. The coding was explained to newcomers and a legend sheet made available to them. A 'general comments' book was kept, principally as a means of communicating between practitioners and to contribute suggestions for improvement. On arrival, the practitioners would peruse the comments to check if there were any pertinent remarks, check the appointment book and prepare the files for the day. Items of general interest, such as notice of seminars, would be posted on the Clinic noticeboard. Finally, an order book for supplies was kept up to date by all.

Collaboration between students and Mission workers was assisted by the Coordinator establishing monthly meetings, some with a lighthearted focus.

Agent A1 reflects:

We functioned as a close team. Meetings were held to discuss the practical issues of rosters, appointments, referrals to facilities and assistance from outside bodies. The task of communicating important messages to other practitioners was a challenging one, particularly as it involved ten or more health workers who had, over the years, developed their own unique notations. It was in response to this challenge that a series of standard symbols was developed to be used by all disciplines.

Agent A2 reflects:

Each month, we would give a presentation to the Mission community about the chiropractic student Clinic. We presented in the "meeting room" which was a place where members of the Mission would gather after lunch. We wanted these presentations to be entertaining as well as informative and welcoming. Chiropractic students variously acted as the chiropractor (comedic name, Dr. McCrack'em) and would present sketches of different patient experiences of a visit to the chiropractor. These role-plays would demonstrate what happened when a person attended the chiropractic Clinic.

Despite these changes, the need for ongoing improvements in communication was recognized. Agent A1 reflects:

More formal training in cultural awareness before students commenced providing services in the Mission Clinic may have led to improvements in collaboration, adaptability and relationship building.

15.4 Critical Reflection: Appreciative Inquiry

Second, critical reflection was undertaken using appreciative inquiry to identify the challenges for collaboration in seeking to replace the habitual practice in health and healthcare of hierarchies. The findings are reported under the headings of the 6Es: Enable, Engage, Enact, Encourage, Evaluate and Emergent (discussed in Chap. 10).

1. Enable

The project was initially enabled by the common commitment of Agent A and the CEO of the NFP Mission to collaborate to provide integrated complementary healthcare for people living in disadvantage. The initial agreement was informal but it was formalized when the university became a collborative partner.

2. Engage
Both the CEO, the two Agents who undertook this reflection and the workers employed by the NFP Mission, were engaged in the design and delivery of the project. Professionals from a range of complementary health specialisms and students were actively engaged in the service provision. Patients were attracted by word-of-mouth to overcome their initial reluctance for hands-on healthcare. The appointment of a clinical co-ordinator by the NFP Mission helped to formalise communication, liasion and organise collaborative meetings.

3. Enact
The NFP provided the physical location for the Clinic. Resources were donated, and over time systems were established to support the Clinic.

4. Encourage
Social networking occurred through formal and informal meetings, and some training was provided.

5. Evaluation
Evaluation of success of the collaboration was not formally undertaken although the ongoing establishment of a Wellness Clinic on site suggests a positive evaluation.

6. Emergence
Emergence of the initial complementary health service provision to a Wellness clinic demonstrates ongoing emergence of the initiative.

15.5 Conclusion

Reflection on the 'Bone Men' project demonstrates, first, the possibility of implementing change from 'the edge' to a more integrated approach to health and healthcare. Second, it highlights the importance of identifying the difference between the project aim and the aim of engaging in a collaborative partnership to achieve the project aim. This was most clearly demonstrated in attempting to evaluate the project. While the Agents were able to demonstrate positive evaluation of the establishment of the Clinic to provide for the health and healthcare needs of the patients, there was no formal evaluation of the effectiveness of the collaborative partnership. For our purpose in seeking to identify what changes are needed in cognition, action to build relationships and action to support a new approach to lead(er)ship in order to achieve a paradigm shift to a holistic ecosystem of health and healthcare, the ecologies and SEERs identified in Chaps. 8, 9 and 10, present a useful means to.

References

Layton Report (1986) Australia, Medicare Benefits Review Committee Report, AGPS, accessible from National Library of Australia, Cat no. 8609346

Marthick-Hone D, Doyle A, Kennedy G et al (2022) The importance of setting and therapeutic relationships when delivering chiropractic care to those living with disadvantage. Chiropr Man Therap 30(1):1–11

Vindigni D (1990) Sacred Heart Mission Heath Programme: experiences of developing a voluntary clinic for the people of St Kilda. Melbourne, Australia, Internal Mimeo Sacred Heart Mission

Chapter 16
Applying Reflection-on-Practice to a Collaborative Pathways to Healthy Ageing: The PHA Project

Dein Vindigni OAM and Sandra Jones

Abstract This chapter presents the findings from applying reflection-on-practice to a health project that was instigated in 2015 as a collaborative partnership. First, a descriptive narrative is combined with concept mapping to explore the project experience of the 3P agencies of health and healthcare. Second, a critical reflection is undertaken, using appreciative inquiry, to identify challenges for collaboration in seeking to replace the habitual practice in health and healthcare of hierarchies of decision making.

16.1 Introduction

The project presented in this chapter was initiated in 2015 as a collaborative partnership between a large Australian university that offers degree qualifications in a range of health disciplines and the CEO of a not-for-profit (NFP) religious and charitable residential aged care facility (RACF) that caters for the local elderly Italian population. The project was initially designed to establish a free-for-service clinic,staffed by university students studying chiropractic, in the grounds of the RACF. After 4 years, students from osteopathy and nursing were also invited to participate. In 2019, the project became part of a larger project established to identify changes needed to extend the experience of the project into a broader approach to Pathways to Healthy Ageing (PHA).

D. Vindigni OAM (✉)
STEM College, RMIT University, Melbourne, VIC, Australia
e-mail: dein.vindigni@rmit.edu.au

S. Jones
Business and Law College, RMIT University, Melbourne, VIC, Australia

S. Jones, D. Vindigni OAM (eds.), *Health and Healthcare in Complexity*,
https://doi.org/10.1007/978-981-96-0515-6_16

The reflection-on-practice in this chapter is undertaken by two agents: the University Chiropractic Discipline leader (B1) and an expert in Complexity science and Distributed Leadership who was engaged as part of a reseach project into the elements of successful collaborative partnerships (B2). First, a descriptive narrative is combined with concept mapping to analyse the experience for each of the 3P agencies of health and healthcare. This is reported in Sect. 16.2. Second, critical reflection is undertaken using appreciative inquiry to identify the challenges for collaboration in seeking to replace the habitual practice of hierarchies in decision making in health and healthcare. This is reported in Sect. 16.3.

16.2 Narrative and Concept Mapping Reflection

16.2.1 Principles and Purposes (P1)

Agent B1 reflects:

My grandmother, Giovanna, became a resident in a Residential Aged Care facility (RACF) in 2015 when she was 92. She already had symptoms of dementia and physical frailty which deteriorated progressively to a point where she was unable to safely be cared for in her own home. After exploring various options, it seemed that a nearby RACF that catered for people from an Italian background would provide the most culturally sensitive and comprehensive care for her needs. As with most people who make the transition from their own homes to residential care, there was an understandable degree of resistance and trepidation which was also shared by her family. The transition brought mixed feelings for all, including a sense of loss from her having to leave her family home, alongside a sense of relief and reassurance that Nonna (grandmother) Giovanna would finally be in a safe and welcoming environment that was sensitive and responsive to her Italian cultural-specific needs. These included the food that she enjoyed, her native language, her Catholic religion, the music that she was familiar with and even some of her long standing friends.

Before her cognitive decline, Nonna Giovanni would often ask me for a neck and shoulder massage which she deeply appreciated. When she stopped communicating verbally, it was clear that she valued the power of touch, often gently squeezing my hand afterwards to express her gratitude. Soon after her transition to the RACF, it became increasingly apparent that tactile therapies of any kind were noticeable by their absence for residents in the RACF.

The value of establishing a collaborative relationship between the RACF and a university that educates students in chiropractic provided the purpose for this project.

Agent B1 reflects:

From my perspective as a clinical specialist and Chiropractic Discipline leader at the partner university, I considered the design of a project based on multiple purposes. First, it could provide a means to respond to research that has identified an increase in the prevalence of chronic musculoskeletal, metabolic and mental health conditions in older people which affect their physical capacity and contribute to an overall decline in quality of life. This research has found that for older people living in RACFs, the adverse effects can be exacerbated by disconnection from their homes and supportive community networks (McCrory et al. 2014). *I also took into account research that has found that, due to the complications imposed by multiple chronic comorbidities, polypharmacy and long-standing opioid and/or sedative use, a more interdisciplinary approach for the attainment of healthy ageing is advocated* (Newhouse and Spring 2010; Fulton and Riley 2005; Hayes et al. 2007). *At the time this project was under consideration, although chiropractic care was available privately in Australia, it was not generally available in RACFs.*

Second, as the academic Discipline Leader of Chiropractic at the university, I was responsible for training new graduates for the chiropractic profession. I believed that providing students of chiropractic the opportunity to gain supervised professional practice experience as part of this project would improve their skills. This approach was supported by the university's Work-Integrated-Learning Policy.

To action the aim, an agreement on both a purpose and a principle, was required.

Agent B1 reflects:

Based in my previous experience in developing a musculoskeletal clinic for people living with disadvantage, I approached the CEO of a local Not–For-Profit [NFP] accredited RACF that is committed to the provision of high-quality, up–to–date, and culturally appropriate services for the Italian community. The chosen RACF provides care for approximately 50 residents who are still able to live relatively independently as their health needs are less critical (i.e. *pre-palliative). Following a presentation to senior managers of the RACF, it was agreed that a clinic would add value to the existing services provided.*

Following the presentation, the CEO agreed to establish a clinic in an open gathering space adjacent to the RACF. A research collaboration agreement (RCA) was signed between the university, the RACF, and the Victorian Branch of the peak professional chiropractic body that was responsible for accreditation of chiropractors.

Agent B1 reflects:

The Project Plan identified the following conditions as necessary for the clinic to function effectively: the provision of a dedicated space for the clinic by the RACF; shared responsibility by the RACF and the university for the provision of staffing, equipment, resources and other facilities; the provision of the services of the RACF Director of Nursing, four Nursing Unit Managers and the resident physiotherapist to assist the clinic; eight staff members and four chiropractic students from the university; funding for the project to be provided by Victorian Branch of the peak professional chiropractic body.

A research plan was designed to evaluate the clinical impacts on the residents and to explore specific clinical issues such as the reliability of a clinical screening tool to screen physical frailty and potentially prevent the risk of falls.

In 2019, a further memo of understanding (MoU) was signed between the university and the RACF to include an expanded number and range of students undertaking professional practice placements and further research.

16.2.2 People in Place (P2)

Recruitment of residents as patients was initially voluntary and opportunistic.

Agent B1 reflects:

It began with some of the more interested or curious residents asking who we were and what we were doing. If there was a language barrier, as a dual English-Italian speaker, I would explain the service to the resident and educate them about the sorts of conditions that might be helped. These included back or neck pain and stiffness, or pain and stiffness in the upper and lower limbs.

Engagement of the RACF staff was encouraged through information and experiential learning opportunities and through the provision of free-for-service chiropractic sessions for them. This had a positive impact as many became regular patients and advocates for the program.

Agent B1 reflects:

Discussions with staff providing existing medical, nursing and physiotherapy care were held to reassure them that the type of chiropractic care that we intended to provide would be personalised, gentle, tailored to residents' levels of frailty, and focused on adding value to existing services.

In response to concerns from the CEO and Director of Care at the RACF as to the level of experience of students, we agreed that initially two students would be chosen. The method of selection was a tiered process that included an expression of interest from applicants, together with my assessment, as their clinical supervisor, of their suitability.

This combination seemed to build bridges of trust and goodwill between the staff, chiropractic students and the chiropractic clinical supervisor.

Feedback from the participants in the initial trial was positive and led to an increase in the number of residents attending the clinic. This led the CEO of the RACF to request an increased number of students to provide services, an extension of student services to include osteopathy and nursing, and an extension of services to residents in higher-level care units who were often socially isolated, lonely, and vulnerable.

Agent B1 reflects:

Overtime, positive feedback was received that the residents would wait for the chiropractic students to arrive and that they commented that the therapeutic touch they offered provided a positive connection.

16.2.3 Practices and Processes (P3)

Given the virtual absence of chiropractic services in RACFs, in the initial project plan, the instigator (Agent B1) designed a series of steps to raise awareness of the contribution that chiropractic services can make to the health and healthcare of residents. Posters and flyers in English were translated into Italian to familiarize residents and families with the (voluntary) opportunity to receive chiropractic service. These were displayed throughout the RACF and emailed to family members of residents (usually the next of kin or medical power of attorney). Existing familial and cultural links between myself and some residents were extended. This meant residents were generally happy to seek treatment and often openly expressed their gratitude.

Agent B1 reflects:

The relatively open and informal nature of the treatment space seemed to invite 'passers-by' to 'come and try' the service. As with establishing clinics of whatever kind, word-of-mouth seemed to be the best source of referral and recruitment of residents.

An initial pilot of the student chiropractic clinic commenced in March 2015. A process was established to roster clinics on Wednesday afternoons from 12.30 pm to 4.30 pm. Treatments mostly included seated neck and shoulder massage therapy as well as knee and foot massage and gentle mobilization, where clinically indicated.

Agent B1 reflects:

Before long, the rapport established between students, the residents and staff became so popular that students were working to capacity. There was no booking of patients as such and though this approach was not likely to be viable in a usual private or community clinic, it seemed to work well in this more informal free-flowing community setting. In time, residents knew that Wednesday afternoons was their day for chiropractic treatment.

Access to electronic patient records by students and the chiropractic supervisor was initially limited to general patient data such as age, room number, and a summary of medical findings and special needs. As trust was built, a system was developed to enable greater student access to patient records. In time, students were able to co-treat residents in their rooms, when required, and with the patient's expressed preference, particularly if residents were frail or limited in their mobility.

Agent B1 reflects:

Over time, the then Director of Care organised for the electronic record-keeping (ERP) system to be programmed so that it allowed for students to enter their patients' notes and to gain greater access to the Medical, Nursing and Physiotherapy clinical findings. Most communication came through electronic records and students also recorded hard copy clinical notes. These were all securely stored in a locked cupboard in the clinic space to which the Nurse Unit Manager and the General Practitioner (GP) had access. Preparation of student hard copy clinical notes and referral letters to the GP, Nursing and other health professionals increased interprofessional dialogue and assisted in the co-management of residents. It also raised awareness of the scope of practice of student chiropractors. Based on these learnings, changes were slowly and progressively integrated to help improve the delivery of the service for both patients and future student cohorts.

However, the building of trust also required significant time to be spent on building relationships.

Agent B1 reflects:

I would informally meet with the visiting GP on occasions to provide updates on developments with the program. This greatly facilitated the exchange of critically important clinical information to better manage, co-manage and refer patients for appropriate treatment.

Regular meetings were held between the student chiropractic clinician, the Director of Care, the CEO, the Nurse Unit Manager, and the physiotherapists, in order to maintain channels of communication. These meetings enabled fine-tuning of the delivery of services.

Agent B1 reflects:

Trained volunteer translators were occasionally made available to assist students in translating information when students were history-taking or explaining their findings. It was also suggested that students participate in a RACF orientation program to familiarise them with the Occupational Health and Safety standards and other policies and procedures of importance. Students seemed to value this opportunity to become acquainted with, and welcomed into, the RACF community.

16.3 Critical Reflection: Appreciative Inquiry

Second, a critical reflection was undertaken using appreciative inquiry to identify the challenges for collaboration in seeking to replace the habitual practice in health and healthcare of hierarchies of decision makings.The findings are reported under the headings of the 6Es: Enable, Engage, Enact, Encourage, Evaluate, Emergent).

1. Enable

The RCA signed by the university and the RACF included standard legal clauses about funding, intellectual property, confidentiality, indemnity and acknowledgement, terms of agreement, and insurance. However, less attention was paid to the details of how to enable collaboration, with clauses limited to general statements on dispute resolution and ethics.

Agent B1 reflects:

This became a problem in 2021 when the CEO left the RACF and I ceased to be the Discipline Leader of Chiropractic. As I was the only person with a detailed understanding of the overarching principles and purpose of the collaboration, the ongoing enactment relied heavily on my knowledge. This challenge was compounded by the growth of the project and the need to maintain relationships for effective collaboration. This all impacted heavily on my time until I received funding from the university in 2019 to conduct research into the collaborative partnerships in developing pathways to healthy ageing.

The challenge was further compounded by the impact of a major external government review into residential aged care that diverted the RACF focus from the expansion of services to the development of measures of the quality of service.

2. Engage

The project was successful in engaging RACF staff, students, and residents and their families in the provision of clinical services to the residents. However, broadening engagment to disciplines beyond medical and allied health service proved challenging.

Agent B1 reflects:

As residents became aware of a more holistic approach to health, they began to ask about the possibility of extending clinical services to establish a Community Garden on the RACF site that would provide them with opportunities for social engagement and exercise. Residents were also excited that this may provide the opportunity to grow typical Italian vegetables and herbs. I held initial discussions with academics from a separate university department (Landscape Architecture) to discuss the opportunity to extend the work-integrated-learning opportunity to students of landscape architecture (to help design a Community Garden). While the initial response from the academics was positive, due to timing issues related to university semesters and a lack of supervisors able to support students, we were unable to progress. A similar challenge was experienced in response to a request from the RACF for a regular program in Tai Chi for the residents. While the university did have a Chinese Medicine Department, students did not have the requisite experience to develop a Tai Chi program for older people.

Despite the setback to planning needed to engage broader groups of students, we were able to use some research project funding to support the engagement of two community groups to establish a 'L'orto dell'Amicizia' (The Garden of Friendship) and to employ an external provider to pilot a Tai Chi program for residents.

3. Enact

The initial enacting of the Clinic staffed by students at the RACF was successful and led to requests to include other allied health (osteopathy) and medical (nursing) services. In turn this resulted in the university decision to fund a research project to design a framework for collaboratIve, integrated pathways to healthy ageing (PHA).

Agent B1 reflects:

I was successful in communicating this knowledge more broadly through an application for an internal university research grant to design a framework for collaborative, integrated pathways to healthy ageing (PHA) based on the experience of this project. However, this highlighted the importance of clearly articulating the link between PAR and evidence-based practice.

An expert in Distributed Leadership was engaged as part of the research project. After an initial presentation on the link between collaboration and Distributed Leadership, a project team was established to oversee the research project.

It adopted a Participatory Action Research (PAR) approach with the aim of collecting feedback to assist the development of a Collaborative Ecosystem for Pathways to Healthy Ageing. The project team met monthly to discuss progress. It relied on feedback from the project team members, students and residents who attended the clinics. The research resulted in the design of a conceptual framework that was endorsed at a forum of representatives from: the university, the RACF, two professional practice bodies (Chiropractic and Chinese Medicine), state and local governments, a healthcare provider, and the University of the Third Age.

Agent B1 reflects:

To embed and sustain the collaboration that had been developed, using the conceptual framework of the Collaborative Ecosystem for Pathways to Healthy Ageing, after the Forum, I established a Pathways to Healthy Ageing (PHA) Community of Interest (CoI) to which I invited representatives from the university, local community groups and local and State government. The PHA CoI continues to meet regularly. Initially, meetings were conducted virtually due to the COVID lockdown, but since 2022, meetings have been face-to-face. It continues to discuss emerging issues and was instrumental in achieving the extension of the initial project into a project to design and deliver a Dementia Awareness and Skills Training program for RACF staff and families of residents. The project is also tasked with preparing a series of Health Promotion Podcasts on Healthy Ageing to promote health, wellbeing, quality of life and social connections for community-dwelling older people.

Agent B1 reflects:

My first step in undertaking this research was serendipitous. I happened upon a meeting with an academic colleague from the College of Business with expertise on the distributed leadership in higher education approach for learning and teaching.[1] *Following this meeting, I proposed that she join the research project as an expert advisor to explore how to underpin the research project with the theoretical framework of a distributed leadership approach that had resulted from her research.*

Subsequently, a facilitated workshop was established to explain how a distributed leadership approach could assist collaboration. The workshop was attended by academic colleagues, the CEO of the RACF, and representatives from interested community bodies.

Agent B2 reflects:

As facilitator of the meeting, I explained the conceptual 6E Distributed Leadership framework that colleagues, and I had developed from research into higher education. Given the positive feedback from participants, we established a Project Team of six members that included four academics, the CEO of the RACF and a representative of a community body that had an interest in improving opportunities for older people (University of the Third Age [U3A]). The project team met monthly for four months to use the experience of the collaboration that had led to and sustained the clinic.

[1] Jones et al. 2012, 2014; Jones 2020, 2017.

In November 2022, following discussions between the incoming CEO, the Director of Nursing of the RACF, senior academic staff from the university School of Health and Biomedical Sciences, and myself, the student clinic was reestablished.

16.4 Conclusion

Reflection on the 'PHA' project demonstrates, first, the possibility of implementing change to a more integrated approach to health and healthcare from 'the edge'. In particular it highlights the advantage of engaging students in an education process that assists them to develop skills for integrated practice (see Chap. 7). Second, it highlights the importance of research into the elements of successful collaborative partnership. In this case the research into collaboration occurred in parallel to the implementation of project. This collaborative research project resulted in the design of a framework for a collaborative ecosystem that was used to achieve broader engagement of experts in discussion concerning issues related to healthy ageing. The authors propose that to embed and sustain future change the ecologies and SEERs identified in Chap. 8, 9 and 10, would provide a useful basis for planning.

References

Fulton MM, Riley AE (2005) Polypharmacy in the elderly: a literature review. J Am Acad Nurse Pract 17(4):123–132

Hayes BD, Klein-Schwartz W, Barrueto F Jr (2007) Polypharmacy and the geriatric patient. Clin Geriatr Med 23(2):371–390

Jones S (2017) Leading the academy: distributed leadership in higher education, HERDSA Guide. HERDSA, Hammondville, NSW

Jones S (2020) Distributed leadership. In: David M, Marilyn J (eds) The SAGE encyclopedia of higher education. SAGE Publications Inc, Thousand Oaks, pp 378–381. Print ISBN: 9781473942912 Online ISBN: 9781529714395

Jones S, Harvey M, Lefoe G, Ryland K (2012) Lessons learnt: identifying synergies in distributed leadership projects: final report. Office for Learning and Teaching. https://ltr.edu.au/resources/LE9_1222_Jones_Report_2012.pdf

Jones S, Hadgraft R, Harvey M, Lefoe, G, Ryland K (2014) Evidence-based benchmarking framework for a distributed leadership approach to capacity building in learning and teaching: final report. Office for Learning and Teaching. https://ltr.edu.au/resources/LE11_2000_Jones_Report_2014_0.pdf

McCrory C, Leahy S, McGarrigle C (2014) What factors are associated with change in older people's quality of life? Tilda, The Irish Longitudinal Study on Ageing. https://tilda.tcd.ie/publications/reports/pdf/w2-key-findings-report/Chapter%206.pdf

Newhouse RP, Spring B (2010) Interdisciplinary evidence-based practice: moving from silos to synergy. Nurs Outlook 58(6):309–317

Chapter 17
Applying Reflection-on-Practice to a Collaborative International Health Hub Rehabilitation Partnership: DHHR Project

Dein Vindigni OAM, Sandra Jones, and Salma Arabi

Abstract This chapter presents the findings from applying reflection-on-practice to a health project that was established in 2021 as an international, cross country, collaborative partnership. First, a descriptive narrative combined with critical incident analysis is used to explore the project experience of the 3P agencies of health and healthcare. Second, a critical reflection is undertaken, using appreciative inquiry, to identify the challenges in seeking to replace the habitual practice of hierarchies of decision making in health and healthcare.

17.1 Introduction

The project presented in this chapter was initiated in 2021 as a collaborative partnership between a large Australian university that offers degree qualifications in a range of health-related disciplines and three nongovernment health providers, each located in one of three lower middle-income countries in the South-East Asian area, Indonesia, Timor-Leste, and Cambodia. The aim of the project, known as the Digital Health Hub Rehabilitation Project [DHHRP], was to design and train in-country health workers to develop their capacity to provide a range of support for people living with pain, impairment, and disability resulting from poor neuromusculoskeletal (bone, joint, muscle, and nerve) health. The three specialisms that the project aimed to integrate were prosthetics, biomechanical therapy, and counselling.

D. Vindigni OAM · S. Arabi
STEM College, RMIT University, Melbourne, VIC, Australia
e-mail: dein.vindigni@rmit.edu.au; sarabi@csu.edu.au

S. Jones (✉)
Business and Law College, RMIT University, Melbourne, VIC, Australia

S. Jones, D. Vindigni OAM (eds.), *Health and Healthcare in Complexity*,
https://doi.org/10.1007/978-981-96-0515-6_17

The reflection-on-practice in this chapter is undertaken by three agents[1]: an Australian-based Director (Relations, Partnerships, and Clinical Education [Agent C1]); an academic expert invited to advise the project team on collaboration using Distributed Leadership (Agent C2), and a PhD student (C3) funded as part of the project. First, a descriptive narrative is combined with concept mapping and critical incident analysis to explore the experience for each of the 3P agencies of health and healthcare. This is reported in S17.2 and 17.3. Second, critical reflection is undertaken using appreciative inquiry to identify the challenges for collaboration in seeking to replace the habitual practice of hierarchies in decision making in health and healthcare. This is reported in 17.4.

17.2 Narrative, Concept Mapping and Critical Incident Analysis

17.2.1 Principles and Purposes (P1)

The DHHRP was influenced by the success of several earlier projects which shared a similar vision of the value of collaborative partnerships between agents in high and middle-income and low middle income countries (LMICs)

Agent C1 reflects:

The project was informed by a project in which I was engaged in 1995 in the Philippines to develop a training program for local people living in a squatter community on a recycling, waste dump (Bagong Barrio). This program included training 80 health workers in basic hands–on-therapies (known as biomechanical therapy) to help address the high burden of musculoskeletal pain and disability experienced in the community.

The DHHRP was conceived in 2020 by three academics in an Australian university with expertise in biomechanics, chiropractic, and clinical psychology. Agent C1 drew on his experience of playing a pivotal role in establishing a previous program in the Philippines.

Agent C1 reflects:

The specific aim of the DHHRP is to develop a training program for health workers in Indonesia, Timor-Leste and Cambodia that integrates Prosthetics, Biomechanical Therapy and Counselling designed to promote the health and wellbeing of people experiencing lower limb loss and/or musculoskeletal pain. The long-term aim is to use the project experience to birth an innovative approach to sustainable health education and healthcare suitable for delivery in LMICs.

[1] The reflections of these three participants are further informed by formal written agreements, meeting notes, and reports.

The project was funded by a global philanthropic body whose aim is to support the development of collaborative partnership to assist LMICs to develop self-sustaining healthcare programs.

A collaborative research agreement (CRA) was signed by the university and the in-country partners. The CRA clarified legal issues of confidentiality, intellectual property, research protocol, and dispute resolution. During the first year of operation, a memo of understanding (MoU) between the Australian university and the CEO of a Canadian-based global not-for-profit (NFP) network was added to enable online clinical materials previously developed for a clinical kinesiology program delivered in Tanzania to be shared. This agreement also linked the DHHRP to a dedicated network of volunteer health professionals able to provide online training assistance.

Agent C1 reflects:

The MOU highlights as its purpose the facilitation of co-operation between the participants for the delivery of the training, without charge, of healthcare and healthcare education in underserviced communities. It highlights the mutual commitments of both parties to consult regularly, share electronic learning resources and learning management systems, and to formally acknowledge the contribution of each. It identifies a dispute resolution process that is based in amicable resolution rather than reference to any external national or international tribunal.

The Canadian NFP also collaborates with ECHO, a worldwide, freely available, online clinical platform in which medical experts volunteer their time to share their knowledge and skills with health professionals caring for under-served communities.

17.2.2 People in Place (P2)

Project leaders from the Australian university and in-country partners were engaged. From the Australian university, two project leaders were employed on a part-time basis, funded by the project. Given the online learning focus, the project was located under the auspices of the inaugural university's Professor of Digital Health as part of the newly established Digital Health Hub. The project leaders consulted with experts from within the university's legal, financial, research, philanthropy, and HR departments. They established teams of experts in the various disciplines and in the design of online education to prepare curriculum material. They also selected a PhD student (funded by the university) to undertake research into the collaborative partnership that underpins the project.

Agent C3 reflects:

As I had recently completed my academic undergraduate degree in the area of educational pedagogy and, as I also had an interest in access and equity to healthcare, I perceived the DHHRP would provide me with the opportunity to pursue a combination of these interests at a post-graduate research level.

Local Not-For Profit (NFP) organizations in-country which had experience in rehabilitation were consulted to identify Project Managers for each in-country partner, to be funded by the project. Following their appointments, the Project Managers in each country employed in-country health practitioners as trainers and local translators and sourced health professionals to become students to be trained in the proffered health techniques. A training stipend was provided for the student health professionals, and funds were allocated from the project to cover the treatment of patients. In-country trainers were first trained (online) as train-the-trainers, by the Australia subject experts. They then used the curriculum material provided to train the student health professionals.

Agent C1 reflects:

From my previous experience of the development of the Sustainable Training, Treatment, Employment Program [STTEP[2]] in the Philippines that had developed as a platform for similar training and had been successfully extended into Cambodia and Indonesia, I was confident that the scaffolded train-the-trainer program would be successful.

17.2.3 Practices and Processes (P3)

The initial project intent was for Australian academic experts to provide face-to-face clinical tuition in each country. Due to travel restrictions imposed by the COVID-19 pandemic, this was changed to online training. This required the design of modules for blended learning that included self-directed, online learning supported by in-country trainers, face-to-face. The formal learning would be reinforced by in-country clinical placements.

Agent C1 reflects:

This suited the philosophy of the global philanthropic funding body as it believed that a blended learning approach had the potential to efficiently increase the reach and impact of clinical skills training programs.

An implementation plan was developed in consultation between the two Australian-based Project Leaders and the in-country Project Managers. The first stage of the project was designed to be implemented in Indonesia in 2021/2022, followed by Timor-Leste in 2022/2023 and Cambodia in early 2023. The plan included the provision of access by in-country partner organizations to the Australian university online learning management system as the platform for delivery of training material. Computer hardware and licenses for software were provided through the grant funding to the in-country partner providers. The original project plan was amended in 2022 to incorporate Indonesian trainers to co-deliver training with in-country partners in Timor-Leste and Cambodia.

[2]Vindigni et al. 2009, 2011.

17.3 Critical Incident Analysis

17.3.1 People in Place (P2): the COVID-19 Pandemic

The first critical incident highlighted the need to ensure that all parties to the collaboration were aware of the details. It involved the delay that occurred in the implementation of the project due to the travel restrictions from the COVID-19 pandemic. This resulted in the loss of some existing contacts that required new networks to be established and new in-country partners to be located.

Agent C1 reflects:

The collaborative partnership was initially formed in 2020 but due to the impact of the COVID-19 pandemic, we lost some of the original partners. This caused me to use my previously established relationships to build new in-country social networks. However, it later became evident that this also led to a loss of understanding of the original principle underpinning the project. This lack of clarity actually contributed to a second critical incident.

While the response was successful, in the short term, in locating new partners, no formal plan was established to cover future contingencies of any loss of relationships. This placed an extra burden of responsibility on Agent C1 to maintain and build relationships rather than have a formalized plan.

17.3.2 Principles and Purpose (P1): New Project Funding

The second critical incident highlighted the need to ensure that there is clear understanding and agreement on the details, and limits, of the collaborative partnership. The critical incident occurred when one of the collaborative partners was successful in their application for funding for a 'spin-off' project to extend training to multiple locations across the country. This was in accord with the national government's strategy to provide similar assistance to other countries in the Southeast Asia region. The funding of the second project resulted in the need to clarify the boundaries of the first collaborative partnership.

Agent C1 reflects:

The successful attraction of further philanthropic funding by our Indonesian partner resulted in the need to clarify the nature of the collaborative partnership. This was resolved through discussion and a new agreement developed that acknowledged the Australian university partner as a secondary partner in the new grant. The new agreement included a commitment to continue to share the university's digital platform and the training material that had been designed.

17.3.3 Practices and Processes (P3) Project Sustainability

The third critical incident highlighted the need to ensure that practices and processes include the development of a sustainability plan. The critical incident occurred at the end of the first year (of a three year funded project) when the philanthropic funding body asked for details on a sustainability plan for the project. During discussion, it became evident that there was no common agreement on what was meant by sustainability.

This led to the need to separate research to evaluate the clinical outcomes of the project from research to evaluate the sustainability of the collaborative partnership. The second research aim was achieved by establishing a joint research team, called the Health Ecosystem Action Relationship for Sustainability (HEARS) team, with representatives from all parties in Indonesia, Timor-Leste, and Cambodia to share reflections of participants on the experience of collaboration in the project.

17.4 Critical Reflection: Appreciative Inquiry

Second, a critical reflection was undertaken using appreciative inquiry to identify the challenges for collaboration in seeking to replace the habitual practice in health and healthcare of hierarchies of decision making. The findings are reported under the headings of the 6Es: Enable, Engage, Enact, Encourage, Evaluate and Emergent (see Chap. 10):

1. Enable

The project initially adopted a conceptual distributed leadership approach to underpin the collaborative partnership between the Australian-based university and the three in-country partners.

Agent C1 reflects:

Having worked previously with an academic expert in the use of a distributed leadership approach to support collaboration, I invited her to help design a strategic plan based on the principles of a distributed leadership framework. The resultant conceptual ecology of distributed leadership for collaborative cross-country partnerships for healthcare is built on the (6E) tenets upon which collaborative partners can self-identify action to: Engage, Enable, Enact, Encourage, Evaluate and support Emergence, and the participation and collaboration of many people.

However, the final formal Agreement did not include a copy of the conceptual distributed leadership framework. This resulted in some confusion about the nature of the decision-making process and of the PhD research aim.

Agent C3 reflects:

There was some initial confusion around whether the primary research focus of the PhD was to be on assessing the development and delivery of the impacts of the train-the-trainer program or on research into collaborative partnerships. As the project unfolded, the focus was clarified as research into the intricate internal dynamics that shape a collaborative partnership's functionality within a broader ecosystem. This clarification reflected a deepening understanding of the importance of identifying the underlying mechanisms and interdependencies that contribute to the effectiveness and sustainability of the partnership. By investigating the intricate layers of collaboration, the PhD aimed to understand how applying an ecological perspective underpinned by a distributed leadership approach may assist in the identification of actions and activities for each party to sustain an international collaborative healthcare partnership.

While a Collaborative Research Agreement (RCA) between the Australian-based university and each of the in-country partners was signed, it was limited to a broad commitment to legalities associated with the partnership rather than providing a detailed guide to the collaborative process.

As discussed in the previous section, it was not until the end of the first year of project implementation that a research design team, termed the Health Ecosystem Action Relationship for Sustainability (HEARS)[3] was established. Its aim was "to develop a strengths-based DHHRP Sustainability Plan built on collaborative principles". It's purpose (agreed by all parties) was to:

(i) Share experience and lessons learned of the four collaborative partners in the initial and ongoing operationalization of the DHHRP project.
(ii) Reflect on these experiences against the 6E action recommendations identified in the conceptual ecosystem of distributed leadership.
(iii) Develop a DHRRP sustainability plan to be communicated to the funding body.
(iv) Develop appropriate milestones and KPIs.
(v) Liaise with the clinical research team.

2. Engage

Parties to the project were identified by the Australian-based Director Operations and the Clinical Education Training Leader and each of the in-country Project Managers. In total, over 51 persons were engaged, 17 by in-country partners and 34 by the Australian partners, in different capacities. Participants were allocated to one of eight groups: an expert group, an expert advisory group (one in each country and a cross-country project team), a scientific committee, and a professional support team.

The HEARS team had a more specific membership consisting of one of the Australian-based Project Directors (Relations; Partnerships and Clinical Education); the in-country Project Managers from the three partner countries; the PhD research student; an expert on Distributed Leadership; and the CEO of a not-for-profit

[3] Internal mimeo from Sandra Jones and Kerryn Butler-Henderson, Head, RMIT Digital Health May 2023.

organisation, Global Peace Network. The HEARS team was supported by a six person expert advisory group.

Agent C2 reflects:

The HEARS team was established with equal representation from each of the collaborative partners. It was underpinned by a reflection-on-Practice approach to encourage members to share their reflections on the future sustainability of the collaborative partnerships.

3. Enact

The project plan was enacted, in the first instance, by one of the Australian-based Director Operations and the Australian-based Clinical Education Training Leader in consultation with the in-country Project Managers. In the first year of implementation, the cross-country project team, chaired by the Director Operations, met regularly to discuss action updates. In-country Project Managers responded to requests for comment. However, the initial findings of the PhD research interviews with the Project Manager in Indonesia revealed a level of deference, based in cultural differences, of the Project Managers to the Director Operations.

Agent C3 reflects:

It became obvious during interviews with in-country project managers in Indonesian that there was a level of deference to the Australian project directors, built on different cultural conceptions of respect. The power appeared to be having a negative impact on open dialogue, as there was hesitancy to question individuals perceived to be "senior" as they held positions of authority. This deference led to responses to research questions about which I raised feelings of unequal contribution within the collaboration.

This was addressed in the second year by the establishment of the HEARS team was established with monthly (digitally suported) meetings during which members discussed lessons learned in accord with the conceptual framework for a distributed leadership approach to the collaborative partnership.

Agent C2 reflects:

In the first year of project operation, discussion on project sustainability was confined to information sharing about what was being achieved. It became clear that there was need to, more definitively, identify what is meant by sustainability. A research team, the Health Ecosystem Action Relationship for Sustainability (HEARS) research design team, was established to focus on research into the sustainability of the collaborative partnership.

4. Encourage

Participation in the project was encouraged by the organizations of biannual workshops held in-country. The second workshop (in Timor-Leste 2023) included a presentation on the conceptual Distributed Leadership ecology. This resulted in its use to explore a potential application for a further grant to embed skills training in Timor-Leste.

Once the HEARS team was established meeting were structured to encourage active participation.

Agent C2 reflects:

While the HEARS research design team is chaired by the Project Director Relations, Partnerships and Clinical Education, facilitation of discussion is encouraged by the preparation and circulation of an agenda which specifies questions to be discussed, prior to meetings, and the circulation of draft Notes after each meeting requesting feedback.

5. Evaluate

Evaluation of the collaboration that occurred in the project was undertaken, in the first instance, through the research being undertaken by the PhD student. The HEARS team established a continual feedback process to evaluate the effectiveness of collaboration. The outcome of the HEARS team was the design of a Framework for the sustainability of the collaborative partnership that was presented to the philanthropic funding body.

6. Emergence

There was evidence of the need for increased attention to be paid to the decision-making process underpinning the project to ensure equal participation by all parties. It was recognised that this would need to pay more attention to the cultural differences in understanding of assumptions related to power.

Agent C3 reflects:

I raised the responses I received in interviews with Indonesian in-country Project Managers as a concern in my PhD supervisor meetings. This led the members of the Australia-based project team to discuss other actions that could be taken to ensure a more culturally aware approach to shared decision-making that would promote greater feelings of equality of contribution by all partners.

17.5 Conclusion

Reflection on the DHHRP, while it demonstrates the potential to implement change to a more collaborative approach, also highlights the detail needed to ensure that collaboration is enabled by formal agreement, that the engagement of people takes account of cultural differences, and that the practice of collaboration is consistent. The authors propose that the ecologies and SEERs identified in Chaps. 8, 9 and 10 would provide a useful framework for future planning.

References

Vindigni D, Polus B, Edgecombe G et al (2009) The STTEP: a model for Musculoskeletal Health Care in Marginalized Communities. J Altern Complement Med 15(8):885–890

Vindigni D, Polus B, van Rotterdam J et al (2011) The sustainable training, treatment, employment program model: effects of manual therapy on musculoskeletal pain and limitation in a Filipino squatter community. J Manip Physiol Ther 34:381–387

Chapter 18
Applying Reflection-on-Practice to a Global Collaborative Transnational Health Training Digital Partnership: THTD Project

Brian Budgell and Sandra Jones

Abstract This chapter presents the findings from applying reflection-on-practice to a global health project that was instigated in the early 2020s in response to the COVID-19 pandemic. It involved a collaborative partnership between a Canadian-based nonprofit charity (Global Peace Network), and a global online training health network (Project Echo). The global collaborative partnership was complicated by the need for GPN to collaborate with existing partners and the government in Tanzania to extend an existing face-to-face training delivery by GPN volunteers in Tanzania. First, a descriptive narrative is combined with concept mapping to explore the project experience of each of the 3P agencies of health and healthcare. Second a critical reflection is undertaken to identify challenges to traditional cultural practices in the recipient country, Tanzania.

18.1 Introduction

The project presented in this chapter was established between a Canadian-base nonprofit charity (Global Peace Network [GPN]) and a global online training network (Project Echo). The project emerged from a 20+ year history of GPN in Tanzania that aimed to improve the health of people living in Tanzania. The on-line project sought to add a digital clinical training platform to the face-to-face training support that had been provided by GPN volunteers. The project is termed the Transnational Health Training Digital Partnership (THTDP).

B. Budgell
Canadian Memorial Chiropractic College, North York, ON, Canada

S. Jones (✉)
Business and Law College, RMIT University, Melbourne, VIC, Australia

S. Jones, D. Vindigni OAM (eds.), *Health and Healthcare in Complexity*,
https://doi.org/10.1007/978-981-96-0515-6_18

The reflection-on-practice in this chapter is undertaken by one agent, the CEO of GPN and an expert in Complexity science and leadership. First, a descriptive narrative is combined with concept mapping to analyze the experience for each of the 3P agencies of health and healthcare. Second, appreciative inquiry is used to identify challenges to traditional cultural practices and to add a critical reflection focus on further design (where do we go from here) and how to empower, learn and adjust for sustainability.

18.2 Narrative and Concept Mapping

18.2.1 Principles and Purposes (P1)

Agent D1 explained that GPN was incorporated as a not-for-profit (NFP) in 2007 to work with local partners to provide healthcare support and education aimed at creating a sustainable model for increased independence. It is focused on implementing holistic projects to improve the livelihoods of impoverished people and their environment. It was initially founded by a young college student with the assistance of a small group of Canadian students who tried to 'do everything, everywhere.'

Agent D1 reflects:

Their approach *included involvement in conserving indigenous music in the Solomon Islands, caring for orphans in the forests of Thailand, and trying to do far too much in Tanzania, including distributing bed nets and food, caring for street-kids and getting involved in health care. It wasn't long before the early members found that they had bitten off more than they could chew, and over time, various projects were wrapped up as the organisation became increasingly focused on addressing musculoskeletal and neurological disabilities and promoting physical rehabilitation.*

The THTDP was designed (or more accurately 'emerged') from recognition of the many musculoskeletal and neurological disabilities that are epidemic in East Africa. The aim is to develop a training program for local health practitioners (including a postgraduate educational program in rehabilitation for government healthcare workers) that incorporates local culture and context. As a result of the impact of COVID-19, it was recognized that the training program needed to be redesigned to incorporate online training using digital transmission.

Neuromusculoskeletal diseases in low to middle income countries, including Sub Saharan Africa, now have the distinction of collectively being the greatest cause of days lost due to disability, and of being a greater burden on national economies than malaria, tuberculosis, HIV/AIDS or all of the cancers combined. Given that approximately half of the citizens of Tanzania (and many other African nations) are younger than 18 years old, this means that there is an enormous population of disabled children. One estimate is that 98% of these children do not attend school, while the World Health Organisation (WHO) (who.int) has stated that perhaps two thirds of childhood disabilities can be effectively mitigated with interventions that are currently available in wealthier countries. By way of example, the prevalence of cerebral palsy in Tanzania is approximately ten times that of its prevalence in Canada. Of course, as may be said of any of us, we only know what we know, and many of our local partners hadno idea how appalling their nation's disability statistics are compared to some other countries.

While it is recognised that there are multifaceted causes of healthcare issues in East Africa, that range from the ergonomics of daily living, inadequate maternal and child-care, and an horrendous neglect of road safety. The project is designed primarily as a digital training program aimed at developing the skills of local health workers in Tanzania to provide rehabilitative care for patients with chronic neuromusculoskeletal diseases/disabilities that are prevalent in Tanzania.

The project accords with the Tanzanian government's aim to modernise health care, as well as the mission of GPN which is to "contribute to a sustainable, hopeful and progressive future for those most impoverished in the world through the development of health care and the provision of education" (globalpeacenetwork.ca).

18.2.2 People in Place (P2)

Tanzania was chosen by GPN because of the high level of chronic neuromusculoskeletal diseases/disabilities coupled with the Tanzanian government's positive support for change.

Agent D1 reflects:

Tanzania is in the late post-colonial stage of development, has a clear national identity and has been a remarkably peaceful and stable country. This is often attributed to Tanzania's first post-colonial president, Julius Nyerere, who promoted nationalism over tribal affinity, combined with the influence of Mahatma Gandhi on Nyerere's thinking. This strong nationalist identity in turn has resulted in progress which, while slow, is enduring. In practical terms, this means that year on year, one sees sustained improvements in roads, schools, hospitals and so forth. All of this, in combination with the remarkable natural beauty and gracious people, make Tanzania attractive both for businesses and philanthropic enterprises.

People are attracted to participate in the project from a place of need rather than being planned. Volunteers provide face-to-face and digital training support.

Agent D1 reflects:

Initially, our (GPN) strategy was quite one-dimensional, focussing on having our clinical volunteers, mostly from Canada and Australia, involved primarily in direct patient care. In fact, while our local partners have considerable expertise in, and have enjoyed success in addressing infectious diseases, they have had essentially no prior training in rehabilitation. However, in response to local in-country feedback that our partners were interested in acquiring the skills of physical rehabilitation, we shifted our emphasis towards the more efficient strategy of educating local practitioners. This turned out to be fortuitous when COVID appeared, as we were obliged to repatriate our volunteers. Now other strategies are in place to sustain our program. These strategies include a digital training program for local practitioners, a digital newsletter and a broad, digitally-based educational hub in partnership with an Australian university.

18.2.3 Practices and Processes (P3)

The strategy for the THTDP project was, firstly, to ensure the ability of local technology to provide access to training. To address the limitations of computer hardware and Internet facilities in Tanzania, the digital training program is accessible through a learning management system (LMS) that allows for the delivery of asynchronous learning modules through a variety of hardware.

Agent D1 reflects:

For example, we found it was unwise to assume that a government office, at any level, would have its own stable internet connection. We experience this, at an amplified level, when meeting with middle managers in District hospitals and health centres where it was unlikely that they would have a working intranet and commonly relied on the staff's personal accounts in order to conduct business. We have therefore found that it is useful to arrive at meetings with a computer and local internet account, and to download, in advance, documents and web pages we might anticipate needing in meetings.

Based on these experiences, we also knew that video conferencing or streaming of audiovisual materials would be challenging. On the other hand, we have found that smartphones, more often vintage versions, are in common usage, with cell coverage surprisingly widespread even if bandwidth is restricted. Accordingly, in developing our online training program, we built upon an LMS that had better functionality and was well suited for smaller and more specialized programs. We designed and developed an entire curriculum for clinical officers and nurses that is compatible with smart phones (which are almost ubiquitous in East Africa), as well as tablets and computers, to permit them to operate as independent providers of physical rehabilitation (posabilities.myabsorb.com). The course of study enables local health professionals to work through the curriculum step-by-step according to their available time.

Experience of technology capacity-issues highlighted the need for ongoing vigilance in the capacity and capability of local technology and Internet connectivity.

Agent D1 reflects:

Despite the attention given to ensuring technological support for digital training, in one of our cases, we found that ECHO sessions were interrupted too often to be useful until we funded a fibre-optic connection to our local hub. Whereas other Project ECHO hubs elsewhere in the world are quite technologically advanced, our own sessions are a bit more modest. Bandwidth does not always allow the use of cameras and connections may drop out. Regardless, we get through our sessions and our local partners really blossom in their clinical behaviours. More recently, we have benefitted from new and growing collaborations; for example, learning resources are being shared with an Australian university.

18.3 Critical Reflection Appreciative Inquiry

Second, a critical reflection was undertaken, using appreciative inquiry to reflect on challenges for habitual cultural practices. The critical reflection uses the 6Es: Engage, Enable, Enact, Encourage, Evaluate, Emergent (see Chap. 10) as a basis for analysis.

1. Enable

The focus of the local Tanzanian partners is on improving healthcare immediately. The challenge is to engage local people in a structured process in accord with the GPN focus on evidence-based care while not wasting time in conducting needs assessments, consulting with stakeholders and developing plans.

Agent D1 reflects:

Our aim of applying an evidence-based approach is an ambitious and worthy aspiration. However, it has seldom been the focus of conversations that we have had with our local partners. Rather, they have consistently focused on how we intend to enact our mission, i.e. *what we are able to do, rather than why. For example, among clinicians, community leaders and patients in more remote locations, the focus is very much on today's needs. Patients, particularly children, suffer and die, absolutely needlessly, and so there is an urgent need to improve health care immediately. Thus, while anyone can understand how repeated individual failures likely reflect systematic failures, individual clinicians, patients and their families are concerned with the here and now. To put an even finer point on that, they want to know what can be done or what they can do, without needing to know why. Thus, evidence-based care, which is often at the core of health care decisions elsewhere, holds little currency in the remote East African community. Our local partners and stakeholders often want to be told what to do. This goes against the grain for many of us trained in wealthier countries, and so we struggle to reconcile the very tangible needs of our stakeholders with the recognition that sustainability can only come through systematic evolution. This particular challenge is augmented by what we might call a cargo-cult mentality at the level of the most local authorities. What I mean by that is the expectation of local bodies is that their role is as recipients of charitable aid, rather than as partners in collaborative development.*

As a consequence, in our discussions and as a matter of course, we have too often found ourselves battling what we might call 'scope creep'—requests or suggestions from our local partners to support projects or organisations which are only most tangentially related to our mission and goals. The positive side of this challenge has been the imperative to bridge the 'why' and the 'what' with a statement of scope which defines what we do within the context of why our organization exists in the first place. This is now front and centre on our website, and we can (and do) point to this as suggestions and requests for assistance come forward.

While such an unstructured approach has led to some successes, it is not advocated, given that there are many examples of a detritus of failed projects in East Africa, including shuttered schools and abandoned clinics, built on the goodwill of well-meaning, but naïve, foreigners.

2. Engage

Traditional Indigenous healthcare is heavily reliant on Ancient Wisdoms that are networked through traditional healers. This means that focus has to be on engaging with traditional healers in a non threatening manner.

Agent D1 reflects:

Let's begin in a very non-digital way with a little introduction to indigenous health care practices in East Africa. Such practices were going through a rough spot when I first visited Tanzania more than a decade ago, due largely to the nefarious behaviours of a few individuals who were not at all representative of the average practitioner. Readers may or may not know that Tanzania has the highest rate of albinism in the world, and, especially in the remote countryside, albinos are both revered and feared for their alleged supernatural powers. One of the outcomes of this was that there was a trade, conducted by self-styled spiritual healers, in the body parts of murdered albinos. Somehow, this led to a wholesale outlawing of indigenous health care practices, although that was soon overturned with the institution of a system of licensing. The government recognized three main sub-disciplines within indigenous medicine. They were herbal medicine, midwifery and what we will call 'bone-setting'. However, every health care practitioner that I have met in Tanzania, whether he/she is a traditional healer, an allied health worker or even an MD, believes in the profound influence of 'spirits' in governing human health. There is no way you are going to get spiritual practices out of the health care system. The lesson for us—a foreign NGO—is that if we are going to 'modernize' the Tanzanian health care system, it is going to be on a different set of terms than we had anticipated.

....And so, one day I was travelling around the countryside in the company of a Tanzanian friend who worked with the local public health authority, liaising with traditional healers. This friend had qualified as a 'clinical officer', which, at that time, required three years of college training after high school. This is the functional equivalent of a medical qualification in other countries, and clinical officers diagnose and treat patients just as medical doctors do elsewhere. This particular friend had also studied abroad and had been in training to become a catholic priest. However, he had been expelled from the priesthood when he found that he could not give up his traditional beliefs. On this day, we visited the home of a traditional healer who subscribed almost entirely to the casting and removal of spells. After he had finished seeing about a dozen patients in the morning, his wives prepared a meal for all of us, including the patients. We sat around a low table in his special treatment hut, dogs and chickens also making themselves at home, and we shared a large plate of ugali—a kind of semi-soft dumpling—and I mean shared with all of the species present, not just the humans. However, before we started to eat, the traditional healer said something in Swahili to my friend. We all bowed our heads, my excommunicated-priest friend said a Christian prayer, everyone said 'amen,' and we waved away the flies and began to eat.

Anyone who has spent any time in East Africa has a chest-full of vignettes, and what many of them illustrate is that there is not one matrix for viewing the world. Where we think we see demarcations between beliefs and practices, others see no such divisions. And, at times, they will see hard barriers where we see none. However, if we—by which I mean outsiders—are going to get along and do some good in these environments, then we have to eat the ugali!

Understanding the close networking that occurs through traditional healers resulted in the recognized need to establish regular communications to develop understanding of different techniques.

Agent D1 reflects:

By focusing on establishing a regular newsletter, we aimed to assist local practitioners to keep up to date with emerging knowledge. A quarterly newsletter, published via *MailChimp (mailchimp.com) and originally targeted at our donors and supporters in Canada, has been adapted and is now also circulated to all of our contacts in East Africa. The newsletter includes summaries of recent and relevant journal or news articles, with hyperlinks to open-access publications. This has the added advantage of, without being overt, nudging our partners towards a shared understanding of our mission and a more evidence-based approach to local health care challenges.*

3. Enact

Ensuring that the local geographical and technological context is understood before seeking to enact change was important. First, the geographical context is highlighted.

Agent D1 reflects:

In addition to the spiritual, much of what has been said about the people with whom we work cannot be separated from the physical and metaphorical, by which I mean cultural, place of Tanzania. East Africa is blessed with valuable minerals, natural gas and vast expanses of arable land, and yet Tanzania is among the poorest countries in the world in terms of gross domestic product per capita. *How could this be? Geography has much to do with the delayed economic development of the country. Most of Tanzania is located on a high plateau which means that river travel into central regions from the coast is not practical. Similarly, the construction of railroads and highways is challenging. Therefore, extraction of resources is impaired and manufacturing enterprises are not attracted to central Tanzania. Abundant rain makes rural roads impassable, or at least difficult to navigate, for several months of the year. Additionally, the tropical climate is conducive to infectious diseases including vector-borne diseases such as malaria. As a practical consequence, it is a routine matter to have projects delayed for weeks or longer because of illness among key stakeholders and partners.*

At each level, if indeed people can be assigned to levels, there are different wants and needs, requiring different approaches. At the governmental level, it is important to recognise that while Tanzania is nominally a democracy, elections and appointments are perhaps more 'managed' that we might experience elsewhere. Consequently, there is probably less urgency to respond to false emergencies and teapot tempests. While it is possible to engage senior politicians and bureaucrats in frank and penetrating discussions, they can take a pragmatic and measured approach to addressing real-world priorities. We (GPN) engaged with representatives of the government at all levels from the Minister of Health to regional and district commissioners, senior politicians and bureaucrats. We also engaged with healthcare practitioners, middle managers in district hospitals and health centres, clinicians, community leaders and patients in various locations.

Second, the technological context:

Agent D1 reflects:

The digitally based education hub was provided through the participation of GPN in a global project operated out of the University of New Mexico (Project ECHO),[1] *Project ECHO is a global project that aims to link clinical experts to local practitioners. We might think of it as grand rounds on electronic steroids. It is hard to keep track of the explosive growth of the ECHO initiative. However, a recent check showed that there were approximately 1000 hubs internationally providing thousands of sessions to millions of participants in almost 200 countries. The technology is simple enough—a Zoom connection (zoom.us)—but the project also provides protocols, teaching resources and the fellowship of like-minded colleagues. At the time of this writing, there are about 90 ECHO programs operating in Africa, which means that the continent is relatively under-represented. However, as internet connectivity improves in leaps and bounds, we expect uptake to soar.*

---

[1] https://hsc.unm.edu/echo/about-us/.

Whereas tele-medicine is modelled on one clinician addressing one patient at a time, Project ECHO is modelled on one expert, or a team of experts, meeting with multiple local clinicians who then go out to care for all of their patients. Therefore, the technology is used to leverage expertise to amplify benefit. The content experts model best practices and the sessions are centered on local practitioners presenting their cases. Data from all of the hubs is collected and analyzed centrally to validate and improve the project. In better-resourced centres, an ECHO session might look more like a movie studio, with elaborate teleconferencing facilities, but great effects can be achieved with far more modest physical facilities.

By adding asynchronous learning through a dedicated LMS, supported by face-to-face clinical training, we have been able to build a resilient, effective program to improve physical rehabilitation in East Africa. (e.g. *the Tanzania Rehabilitation Initiative). This has added value over the 15 years of our transnational partnership in Tanzania. We have constructed a couple of rehabilitation clinics and brought in volunteers to treat patients and teach local practitioners while at the same time making strong efforts to be respectful of local, including traditional, health care practices. Digital technologies have proven invaluable in all of this, by contributing much to addressing the challenges of developing a shared purpose and a robust theoretical framework for action.*

18.4 Conclusion

Reflection on the THTDP demonstrates the possibility of implementing change in projects 'from the edge'. However the findings also demonstrate the central importance of taking into account traditional Principles and Purpose (P1), engaging with local traditional healers (People in Place [P2]) and designing Practices and Processes (P3) that not only take into account local habitual social and spiritual culture but also the geographic and technological context. Second, this project highlights the need to clearly identify a plan to support and sustain collaboration. For our purpose in seeking to identify what changes are needed to achieve a paradigm shift to a holistic ecosystem of health and healthcare, the ecologies and SEERs identified in Chaps. 8, 9 and 10 could provide a valuable framework for collaboration and collaborative partnerships.

Chapter 19
Applying Reflection-on-Practice to a Collaborative Indigenous (Aboriginal) Health Hands-on-Health Initiative: AHAH1 Project

Dein Vindigni OAM and Sandra Jones

Abstract This chapter presents the findings from applying reflection-on-practice to an Indigenous heath project that was established in 1998 as a collaborative initiative between a university and two Indigenous organizations in Australia. First, a descriptive narrative is combined with concept mapping to explore the potential relationship between the 6Ls of Australian Indigenous Ancient Indigenous Wisdoms and the 3P agencies of the holistic ecosystem of health and healthcare. Second, a critical reflection is undertaken using appreciative inquiry to identify a potential relationship between the factors that contribute to a holistic ecosystem of health and healthcare and Ancient Indigenous Wisdoms.

19.1 Introduction

The project presented in this chapter was undertaken in 1998 as a collaborative initiative between an Australian university (a School of Medical Practice and Population Health) and two Indigenous organizations (the Durri Aboriginal Health Service (DAHS) and the Booroongen Djugun Aboriginal Health College). The project was titled 'Promoting the Musculoskeletal Health of Indigenous Australians Living in Rural Communities: Aboriginal Health in Aboriginal Hands' (termed

D. Vindigni OAM (✉)
STEM College, RMIT University, Melbourne, VIC, Australia
e-mail: dein.vindigni@rmit.edu.au

S. Jones
Business and Law College, RMIT University, Melbourne, VIC, Australia

S. Jones, D. Vindigni OAM (eds.), *Health and Healthcare in Complexity*,
https://doi.org/10.1007/978-981-96-0515-6_19

AHAH1 for the purpose of this book[1]). The aim of the project was to develop and implement a community-based musculoskeletal health training program for Indigenous Australians living in a large rural community in New South Wales. This was part of a broader initiative to help inform culturally sensitive musculoskeletal health promotion strategies. The project involved the addition of Western complementary (chiropratic) healthcare to an Indigenous approach.

The reflection-on-practice in this chapter is undertaken by one of the (people) agents, who was then a PhD candidate in the School of Medical Practice and Population Health at the Australian university. First, a descriptive Narrative combined with concept mapping is used to explore a potential relationship between the 6Ls of Ancient Indigenous Wisdoms (see Chap. 12) and the 3P agencies of the holistic ecosystem of health and healthcare. Second, a critical reflection is undertaken, using appreciative inquiry, to explore any potential relationship between the factors contributing to a (Western) holistic ecosystem of health and healthcare and the Ancient Indigenous Wisdoms.

19.2 Narrative Reflection

19.2.1 Lore and Love (L1 and L2) and Principles and Purposes (P1)

The Aboriginal Health in Aboriginal Hands (AHAH1) project was influenced by two key principles and purposes: first, the importance of providing palliative care to people living with disadvantage and, second, the desire to promote the musculoskeletal health of Indigenous Australians living in rural communities.

Agent EI reflects:

> I *was influenced by the experience, as an Australian participant on an Australian Community Aid Abroad Trip to India in the 1980s, visiting various humanitarian projects being including establishing volunteer-run clinics to provide healthcare to people who lived in slum areas in Calcutta and a community development project to assist bonded labourers to establish communal crops to help break the cycle of poverty. During this trip I was privileged to meet several inspiring humanitarians, Ms Moira Kelly and Satish who had left New Delhi to move to a poor rural village in Uttar Pradesh. Satish worked closely with bonded labourers who had inherited dowries which often took a lifetime to pay after accepting loans from wealthy non-tribal landowners. Satish and his helpers established a community-development project in which bonded labourers pooled their seedlings, grow and harvest communal crops and share the earnings to help pay back the loans and help break the cycle of poverty.*

[1]The outcome of this project was the establishment of an ongoing project termed Indigenous Health in Indigenous Hands (AHAH) under the auspices of Hands on Health Australia (HOHA). To indicate the separation between the project discussed in this chapter and the ongoing AHAH, the term AHAH1 is used in this chapter.

Satish mused about our trip to India. Though he expressed gratitude for our team's visit and willingness to listen and learn about this community development initiative, he was aware of the great poverty created by homelessness, loneliness, mental illness and poverty of spirit in the Western world which further contributed leads to a downward spiral of suffering and ill health. Satish encouraged us to reflect on these other faces of spiritual poverty in our own 'back yards', a poverty which, though hidden at times, were just as real and often even more difficult to address.

It was in a multidisciplinary clinic in Newcastle in which I worked as a chiropractor in the 1990s that I first learned about Uncle Paul Gordon, through a patient who would regularly meet with him at Wollombi, a sacred area of the Awabakal people, the Traditional Custodians of this Community. I attended a small cultural gathering at Wollombi. We sat around a campfire and shared stories about our life journeys, traditions as well as challenges, hopes and dreams. This included discussion about the importance of traditional Ancient Indigenous Wisdoms, especially of looking, listening and learning from each other. We shared stories about traditional Indigenous and other hands-on healing approaches. Subsequent cultural gatherings and meetings revealed other Ancient Indigenous Wisdoms.

19.2.2 Look (L3) and Listen (L4) and People in Place (P2)

Two further Ancient Indigenous wisdoms were demonstrated during subsequent meetings in which there was a sharing of knowledge about the application of Indigenous and allied and complementary therapies. This led to the emergence of the idea for a joint project in which both approaches and ideas could be shared. This is in keeping with the common message in Aboriginal spirituality of the importance of Looking, Listening, and Learning from each other wherever we come from or whatever our beliefs are.

Agent E1 reflects:

Uncle Paul Gordon emphasises the importance of sharing the gifts of Creation more fairly, to nurture each other and the land which, like an umbilical cord, sustains us. During many meetings Uncle Paul spoke of the foods, fibres and medicines of the Awabakal people and Ngemba people (of New South Wales-NSW) and Ancient stories and Wisdoms of his Elders. He reflected on the importance of Country as teacher and healer, stating: the bush is our supermarket, hospital, gym and Church. It provides for all of our needs which is why we embrace Ngurampaa...which, in Ngemba means – I love my place and everything in my place.

As a chiropractor, my hands are my main tool and Uncle Paul was interested in learning some of our techniques such as trigger point therapy (similar to acupressure) for alleviating pain and disability. We reflected on the synergies between traditional, Indigenous approaches to healing and Allied and Complementary therapies such as chiropractic, osteopathy, Chinese medicine and myotherapy. and people of like-heart regardless of their background, working together to bring renewed hope and healing to all.

The outcome was the decision to establish a joint collaborative project between a local university and a local Indigenous community advisory group.

19.2.3 Learn (L5) and Lead (L6) (or Leave Alone) and Practices and Processes (P3)

The project itself was preceded by informal training of Aboriginal health workers in simple massage techniques during these cultural gatherings. The purpose was to demonstrate how to help alleviate the chronic pain and impairment endured by so many community members who lacked the funds and access to even basic medical services. Based on this experience, the project was designed to be underpinned by a PhD research project using a Participatory Action Research approach to capture the living nature of Ancient Indigenous wisdoms. First, a survey was undertaken to document the pain and disability experienced by Indigenous Australians in 'the bush' as the first step to inform culturally sensitive musculoskeletal health promotion strategies. Second, findings from the initial survey and clinical assessments were used to inform the design, development, and delivery of a community-based musculoskeletal health training program for the community. This was to be underpinned by the bilateral exchanges of knowledge that included basic, traditional Indigenous approaches to healing (including bush foods and medicines) and hands-on healing techniques such as sports massage, stretching, strengthening, and exercise. Sports massage was suggested as a culturally suitable therapy for training members of the community, given the importance of sport in bringing community together on 'common ground.'

Agent E1 reflects:

Uncle Paul Gordon believes that in order to promote the health and wellbeing of Aboriginal and non-Aboriginal people, we need to speak a common language understood by healers, decision-makers and politicians including evidence of the health problems and practical, sustainable solutions that address these health problems. It was inspired by Uncle Paul's vision to take small steps towards bringing about renewed hope and healing for all people in this country.

This led to my enrolling in a PhD titled "Promoting the musculoskeletal health of Indigenous Australians living in rural Communities: Aboriginal Health in Aboriginal Hands, which was completed in 2004.

19.3 Appreciative Inquiry

A second reflection was undertaken using appreciative inquiry to identify any potential relationship between the 6Es of a holistic ecosystem of health and healthcare (see Chap. 10) and the 6Ls of Ancient Indigenous Wisdoms. The findings are explained below.

19.3.1 Lore and Enable

The project was underpinned by the embracing of Ancient Indigenous Wisdom encapsulated by the 6Ls (Lore, Love, Look, Listen, Learn, Lead [or Leave alone]).[2]

Agent E1 reflects:

From the beginning Uncle Paul encouraged interested health professionals to learn more about the richness of traditional Aboriginal approaches to healing and, together, to take steps towards understanding and managing the pain and suffering endured by the Community.

Elders and the Board of Directors at the Aboriginal Corporation Health Service (ACHS) endorsed the musculoskeletal prevalence study that informed the pilot Sports massage course, which would act as a model for training Aboriginal Health Workers (AHWs) in the culturally appropriate assessment and management of common musculoskeletal conditions affecting their people.

To gain ethics consent from the university, the Board of Directors from the ACHS reviewed the protocol for the study and liaised with various representatives from the Community to determine the cultural acceptability of the study. These representatives contributed significantly to the development and review of the project and assumed the role of the Community Advisory Group (CAG). The university subsequently accepted the proposal as meeting university protocols.

19.3.2 Love and Engage

A broad representation of Indigenous Elders, community groups, health workers, and patients was included in the design and establishment of the project.

Agent E1 reflects:

In keeping with Uncle Paul's approach of drawing from the collective wisdom of the Community to inform collaborative solutions, a CAG was established, to ensure that the project remained sensitive and genuinely responsive to the needs of the Community. The Board of Directors from the Aboriginal Community Health Service (ACHS) participated in the CAG, alongside Elders, Aboriginal Health Workers (AHWs), patients from the ACHS and the PhD researcher. Also included were representatives of a remote branch of the ACHS, the two main Community drop-in centres, the retirement centre and an Indigenous aged care centre.

In addition, an Aboriginal healthcare training college, a local university and a not-for profit healthcare organisation.

Members of the CAG had a deep understanding of where younger and older members of the Community could be more readily reached to enable a cross-section of the Community to be recruited.

[2] See Chap. 12.

19.3.3 Look and Enact

The project was enacted through a series of phases, a preparation phase, a research phase, and an implementation phase, during which the community's needs were identified, actions designed, and systems of support implemented.

Agent E1 reflects:

Phase 1 commenced with chiropractors, osteopaths and massage therapists who visited the Community twice yearly and conducted small workshops in massage in the Aboriginal Medical Service (AMS) as well as providing tactile therapies to the Community.

Phase 2 involved a cross-sectional survey of the local Indigenous Community to identify the prevalence of musculoskeletal condition, and an assessment of the associated risk factors and barriers to managing these conditions in the Community The results were validated by a clinical assessment.

Phase 3 involved the co-design pilot and implementation of a Community-based musculoskeletal health promotion program, termed Aboriginal Health in Aboriginal Hands (AHAH) delivered by AHWs.

The AHAH program attempted to incorporate both identifying modifiable risk factors (to facilitate the prevention of musculoskeletal conditions) and opportunities for managing the most prevalent musculoskeletal conditions, primarily in the form of, massage therapies and self-help strategies such as stretching and strengthening exercises as well as the documentation and sharing of some traditional approaches to healing including bush medicines as taught by Elders of the Community.

On average, the CAG met every month, usually at the Aboriginal Health Service in Kempsey (Dunghutti Country, NSW), and in smaller groups in between times when needed.

19.3.4 Listen and Encourage

Ongoing participation in the project was encouraged by guidance from members of the CAG who proposed and helped establish Community engagement sessions.

Agent E1 reflects:

This project resulted from much listening to the embedded wisdom in the stories of Elders, members of the Community and Indigenous and non-Indigenous collaborators, including health professionals, academics and researchers.

Through activities, such as welcoming focus groups run as yarning sessions and implementing suggestions for change as they arose, we continued to build engagement. One important change included the incorporation of traditional, Indigenous approaches to healing.

19.3.5 Learn and Evaluate

The project was positively assessed as acknowledging cultural sensitivities by incorporating Indigenous approaches in the management of musculoskeletal conditions. It also affirmed the value that the Community attached to sport. Importantly, the AHAH was shown to be a culturally acceptable step toward promoting the musculoskeletal health of Indigenous people living in this rural Community.

19.3.6 Lead or Leave Alone and Emergence

The project has a sustained impact both for initial graduates of the program and has since been developed into an allied health program for other members of Community.[3]

Agent E1 reflects:

Recommendations from the project as a sustainable, Community-based training initiative to help improve the musculoskeletal health of Indigenous Australians included: i) priority for cultural sensitivity and collaboration to underpin planning of health service delivery with and for Indigenous people; ii) a Community-based model to be seeded in Communities throughout the country as a step towards promoting the musculoskeletal health of Indigenous people living in rural Australia and beyond.

Several Aboriginal Health Worker graduates from the original AHAH program delivered in the Community continue to integrate the learnings from the program in their various roles in Community sporting events, aged care and health promotion initiatives carried out in the Aboriginal Community Health Service and its outreach services.

This AHAH program is currently being delivered to First Nations allied health students and other members of the Community and its impact being delivered via *a co-design process.*

19.4 Conclusion

Findings from the application of the reflection techniques of narrative, concept mapping and appreciative inquiry demonstrate the possibility of a holistic ecosystem of health and healthcare being extended to acknowledge and include Ancient Indigenous Wisdoms. However, before this can be achieved, there is need for further consideration of the Spiritual that underpins Ancient Indigenous Wisdoms. The authors propose that the Holistic Spiritual Inclusive Ecosystem (HSIE) and SEER S identified in Chap. 13 could provide a valuable framework for further research.

---

[3] See references.

References

Doyle KE, Zarb L, Wilkey K, Sale K, Pitt C, Vindigni D (2020) Embedding cultural competence in faculty: a mixed-methods evaluation of an Applied Indigenous Proficiency Workshop. In: Cultural competence and the higher education sector: Australian perspectives, policies and practice. Springer, pp 277–293

Polus BI, Paterson C, Van Rotterdam J, Vindigni D (2012) Embedding chiropractic in Indigenous Health Care Organisations: applying the normalisation process model. BMC Health Serv Res 12:1–9

Vindigni D, Parkinson L, Rivett D, Da Costa C, Perkins J, Walker BF, Blunden S (2006) Developing a musculo-skeletal screening survey for Indigenous Australians living in rural communities. Rural Remote Health 6(1):1–14

Vindigni D (2005) Promoting the musculoskeletal health of Indigenous Australians living in rural Communities. Aboriginal health in aboriginal hands [PhD]. University of Newcastle, Newcastle

Vindigni D, Parkinson L, Walker B, Rivett DA, Blunden S, Perkins J (2005b) A community-based sports massage course for Aboriginal health workers. Aust J Rural Health 13(2):111

Vindigni D, Walker BF, Jamison JR, Da Costa C, Parkinson L, Blunden S (2005a) Low back pain risk factors in a large rural Australian Aboriginal community. An opportunity for managing co-morbidities? Chiropr Osteopat 13:1–12

Vindigni D, Griffen D, Perkins J, Da Costa C, Parkinson L (2004a) Prevalence of musculoskeletal conditions, associated pain and disability and the barriers to managing these conditions in a rural, Australian Aboriginal community. Rural Remote Health 4(3):1–13

Vindigni DR, Parkinson L, Blunden S, Perkins J, Rivett DA, Walker BF (2004b) Aboriginal health in Aboriginal hands: development, delivery and evaluation of a training programme for Aboriginal health workers to promote the musculoskeletal health of Indigenous people living in a rural community. Rural Remote Health 4(4):1–10

Part IV
Implementing Change for Health and Healthcare: Learning Through Doing

Part IV of this book returns to the aim identified in Chap. 1 of seeking to provide not merely an argument for a change to health and healthcare, but to assist those who acknowledge the need for such a change to self-identify actions appropriate to their context and culture. The purpose of Part IV is to revisit the four Self Enabling Ecologies of Reflection (SEERs) that we created from our reflections in Chaps. 8, 9, 10 and 13 to suggest how those wishing to engage in change towards a holistic ecosystem of health and healthcare can self-identify actions appropriate to their context and culture.

Chapter 20
Using the Self Enabling Ecologies of Reflection

Sandra Jones

Abstract The aim of this chapter is to assist those who acknowledge the need for a shift in paradigm to a holistic ecosystem of health and healthcare to self-identify actions appropriate to their context and culture.

20.1 Introduction

In Chap. 1 of this book, we stated that our aim is not merely to present an argument for change to health and healthcare but to assist those who acknowledge the need for change to self-identify actions appropriate to their context and culture. We likened our approach to that of *wayfaring*, which is made up of three parts. First, through *wayfinding*, or navigating, observing and identifying likeness and systems. We presented this in Part I as the challenges health and healthcare built on principles of Cartesian science when operating in the current world of complexity. Second, through *wayshowing*, or trailblazing, leaving clues, planning and creating new directions. We presented this in Part II with our discussions and reflections leading us to the assemblage of four ecologies that together contribute to a holistic ecosystem of health and healthcare. The ecologies were designed to underpin collaboration through changes in cognition (the Collaborative Adaptive Resilient Ecology [CARE] in Chap. 8), in actions to build relationships (the Distributive Action Relational Ecology [DARE] in Chap. 9), and in a new form of lead(er)ship (the Lead(er)ship Ecology of Adaptive Practice [LEAP] in Chap. 10). Assembled together we identified an integrated Action Cognition Ecology of Leadership [ACEL] in Chap. 10. Finally, we assembled an ecology designed to recognise the spirit of Indigenous living (in addition to the mind–body emphasis of Western

S. Jones (✉)
Business and Law College, RMIT University, Melbourne, VIC, Australia

S. Jones, D. Vindigni OAM (eds.), *Health and Healthcare in Complexity*,
https://doi.org/10.1007/978-981-96-0515-6_20

thinking) into what we termed a Holistic Spiritual Inclusive Ecosystem (HSIE in Chap. 13). Alongside these ecologies, we created resources in the form of Templates of Self Enabling Ecologies of Reflection (SEERs) to enable individuals and groups who acknowledge the need for change to self-identify actions appropriate to their culture and context. Third, through *waysharing*, or storytelling, we transferred information, through sensemaking and consciously evolving. This we presented in Part III as the findings from reflection-on-practice of five projects that sought to achieve change to a more integrated health and healthcare through collaboration.

Our aim in Part IV is to suggest steps for individuals and groups to plan and implement action to achieve collaboration designed to assist the paradigm shift to a holistic ecosystem of health and healthcare. To do this, we revisit the self-enabling ecologies of reflection and explain how they can be used to facilitate self-determination of actions through self-reflection.

20.2 The Self-Enabling Ecologies of Reflection (SEER)[1]

The Self-Enabling Ecologies of Reflection (SEER) were created as resources to assist individuals and groups to self-identify opportunities to design activities to assist implementation of changes in: cognition (SEER C); methods of action to build relationships (SEER A); approach to lead(er)ship (SEER L); and to include the spiritual; in a holistic ecosystem of health and healthcare (SEER S). The SEERs are designed with the following features:

1. Each acknowledge the 3Ps agencies of health and healthcare: Principles and Purposes (P1), People in Place (P2), and Practices and Processes (P3).
2. SEER C is designed to assist reflection on the contribution of the 3P agencies to plan for, and implement, change to modes of cognition. We acknowledged in Part II four modes of cognition: systems thinking, sensemaking, reflective thinking and social ecological thinking.
3. SEER A is designed to assist reflection on the contribution of the 3P agencies to design and implement actions to build relationships. We acknowledged in Part II four methods of action: distributive engagement, social networking, participative action research and reflexive practice.
4. SEER L is designed to assist reflection on change to encourage a more collaborative form of lead(er)ship. We acknowledged in Part II three forms of leadership, which we later considered to be explained by the 6 tenets of Distributed Leadership (Engage, Enable, Enact, Encourage, Evaluate and Emergence).
5. SEER S is designed to assist reflection on change designed to acknowledge the spiritual in Indigenous lives.

[1] The SEERs are consolidated at the end of this chapter.

20.3 Using the SEERs to Plan for, and Implement, Change to a Holistic Ecosystem of Health and Healthcare

As discussed earlier, in recognition of the extent of change required, and in acknowledgment that those embedded in the current paradigm will be less committed to change, our proposal is for change to be implemented from 'the edge'. We demonstrated in Parts II and III that this can be achieved through a distributive approach based on projects and project teams who employ research techniques that engage many experts in cycles of change. However, we also identified that proposals for collaboration, within and between teams and partnerships, are scarce on details of how project teams can function, apart from acknowledging the advantage of Participatory Action Research and Reflection. Our proposal is for project teams to be guided by the reflection prompts outlined in the four SEERs as follows. The sequence of these steps may vary according to context and culture.

1. Once a project has been identified, consider what expertise is needed and who can be *engaged* to provide that expertise (People in Place [P2]).
2. Once established ensure that to *enable* the project team to function effectively, there is an agreed aim (of collaboration), (Principles and Purpose [P1]). At this point, it is important to acknowledge that the project team will have two foci: (i) the identified project aim and (ii) effective collaboration to achieve this project aim. For example, in the projects discussed in Part III, it was identified that there were two aims acting together: (i) the aim of integrating types and forms of health expertise to address the health issues of the patients and (ii) the aim of designing and implementing the project as a collaborative partnership.
3. Discuss what Practices and Processes (P3) are needed to *enact* the project and to *encourage* and support the team (this may include systems, technology, finance, training, time allocation).
4. Agree what methods of *evaluation* you intend to use. Once again the importance of developing two forms of assessment is highlighted: (i) to evaluate progress towards the project aim and (ii) to evaluate the effectiveness (and possible sustainability) of the collaboration.
5. It is at this point that the choice, and sequence, of the SEERs is important. This requires consideration by the team of whether a change in cognition (SEER C); action to build relationships (SEER A), lead(er)ship (SEER L); or consideration of the spiritual (SEER S) to achieve a holistic ecosystem is of most importance in the specific context and culture.
6. Once the appropriate SEER is chosen, follow the reflective prompts identified in the SEER templates and record the responses of all engaged in the project.
7. If there are differences of opinion, discuss these, with the aim of coming to an agreement that is formally recorded (and signed by all relevant people if appropriate). If at this stage it is found that there is not a commonly agreed process to address differences and negotiate agreement, this may need clarification (and perhaps formal agreement).

8. Build into the planning of the project time for reflection (reflection points) for observation, feedback, clarification, and change as the project unfolds. This enables consideration of the dynamic nature of the project. It may require additional funding, training, systems of communication and changes to timetables.
9. At the end of the project build in a formal time to reflect on the effectiveness of collaboration within and between project team members (and outside experts). These reflection points, both during or at the end of the project, can be used to encourage the design of change to underpin a further cycle for the project.

20.4 Final Words

As authors, practitioners and researcher committed to the need for a paradigm shift to a holistic ecosystem of health and healthcare, we trust that we have provided food for thought and action by those who *dare to care* to implement change to address the complex challenges facing humanity.

Template 8.1 Self-Enabling Ecology of Reflection on Cognition (SEER C)

Use the reflection prompts to identify changes in cognition associated with each of the modes of thinking…

3P agencies of health and healthcare	Systems thinking	Sensemaking	Reflective thinking	Social ecological thinking
P1 **Principles and purposes** *systems, relations and interconnections*	*…encourage understanding of the organisation as a whole*	*…encourage the unfolding and emergence of new systems*	*…focus on emergence of solutions based on lessons learnt*	*…encourage understanding of dynamic interconnections between all agencies*
P2 **People in place** *agents who collaborate and co-evolve through interactions, relationships, self-organisation and diversity*	*…enable relationships between elements to seek future order arising from complexity*	*…enact collaborative, reciprocal relationships*	*…encourage reflection beyond the individual to the collective*	*…engage professionals, patients, families and communities*
P3 **Practices and processes** *spontaneous emergence of order, structure, stability and adaptability*	*…enact interdependent microsystems that are embedded at multiple levels*	*…encourage circumstances to be turned into situations as springboards to action*	*…create and clarify meaning through critical reflection*	*…collaborate to achieve a holistic approach to public health*
interactions through feedback loops and information sharing	*…encourage non-linear thinking*	*…evaluate performativity of practice*	*…evaluate inclusive of human agency and culture*	*…encourage integration between separated professions*
external factors (training, finance, public attitude)	*…encourage "living with" unpredictable and uncontrollable elements*	*…encourage thinking based on ecological change*	*…critically reflect on self in relation to self, and to the world*	*…mix clinical (technical) and individual (lived) experience*
knowledge growth and team behaviour	*…encourage open communication in ambiguity, uncertainty, disorder or chaos*	*…focus on emergent patterns*	*…enable new knowledge through retrospective contemplation of practice*	*…encourage acceptance of emergence (rather than blame) to shape and develop futures*

Template 9.1 Self-Enabling Ecology of Reflection on Action (SEER A)

Use the reflection prompts to identify changes in action to build relationships associated with each of the methods of action…

3P agencies of health and healthcare	Distributive engagement	Social networking	Participatory action research	Reflexive practice
P1 **Principles and purposes** *Collaboration*	*…enable identification of a common principle through top-down, bottom-up and middle-out and*	*…enact understanding of social systems as a source of collaboration for new ideas and practice*	*…enact action and research to occur in concert for collaboration between participants engaged in empirical change*	*…encourage collaboration through knowing based in doing*
P2 **People in place** *Interrelated*	*…encourage cross-sector, cross-discipline and multi-level interrelationship engagement*	*…encourage identification of nodes and the linked relationships between them*	*…encourage participation and research in interrelated teams engaged in empirical cooperative inquiry*	*…enact dynamic change through appreciation of the interrelationships between knowing and doing*
P3 **Practices and processes** *Interconnected*	*…encourage bi-directional inter-communication and networking*	*…encourage interconnections through communication and information flows between nodes (people, objects and associations)*	*…encourage problem-solving for emergence as part of EBP through interconnected cycles to develop innovations*	*…enact simultaneous thinking and practice*

Template 10.1 Self-Enabling Ecology of Reflection on Lead(er)ship (SEER L)

Use the reflection prompts to identify changes to acknowledge lead(er)ship as an activity

3P agencies of health and healthcare	*…ENABLE…*	*…ENGAGE…*	*…ENACT…*	*…ENCOURAGE…*	*…EVALUATE…*	*…FOSTER EMERGENCE…*
P1 Principles and purposes	*…the work of lead(er)ship*	*…in relationships based on values of inclusivity and diversity*	*…collaboration as part of a collective*	*…understanding of lead(er)ship*	*…by identifying means to demonstrate outcomes against aims*	
P2 People in place	*…alignment of personal and professional values*	*…people with expertise, interest, time and funding*	*…a coalition of the willing with perseverance and commitment to intellectual growth*	*…awareness and understanding of collaboration …curiosity, an open mindset and communication for understanding*	*…by adding measures of enjoyment and alignment of values*	*…by creating conditions for serendipity*
P3 Practices and processes (i) Systems	*…the balancing of autocracy and democracy*	*…diverse individuals by actions to…*	*…the design of systems for conflict resolution to prepare participants to work together*	*…two-way communication and understanding*	*…by identifying impact through stories*	*…by implementing cycles of change*
(ii) Processes	*…living with uncertainty*	*…in processes to maintain momentum over time*	*…collaboration in relationships*	*…structural support to build resilience*	*…by recognising and rewarding contribution*	*…by attracting ongoing cumulative funding*

Template 13.1 Self-Enabling Ecology of Reflection on Spirit (SEER S)

Use the reflection prompts to identify examples of the conjoining of Western (3P agencies) and Indigenous approach to cognition…

3P agencies of health and healthcare	LORE (1)	*Ancient* LOVE (2)	*Indigenous* LOOK (3)	*Wisdoms* LISTEN (4)	LEARN (5)	LEAD (OR LEAVE ALONE (L6)
Principles and purposes (P1) *…encourage understanding of the organisation as a whole*	*…Ancient knowledge as wisdoms required to live in harmony with all creation*	*…respect for Indigenous spiritual and cultural practices*	*…awaken perceptive capacities to notice and observe Earth-Kin*	*…share the gifts of creation*	*…contentment comes from finding meaning and purpose through learning and growth*	*…achieve the best outcome for all through establishing relationships with people and Country*
People in place (P2) *…enable collaborative, reciprocal relationships*		*…relationships built in good intentions and motivations*	***…**people actively watch and observe nature (bush)*	*…gain knowledge by looking and listening*	*…engage in community through learn through cultural respect and community*	*…engage humans in balance with nature*
Practices and processes (P3) ***…**encourage interdependent systems to clarify meaning and springboard collaborative action*	*…Ancient knowledge as wisdoms required to live in harmony with each other*	*…encourage exchange of stories*	*…observe and begin to appreciate acceptable (and unacceptable) practices*	*…listen with humility respect and patience to individual stories*	*…look and listen to gain understanding of local culture knowledge*	*…design teaching and learning that is locally oriented, & designed to restore ecological balance*

GPSR Compliance

The European Union's (EU) General Product Safety Regulation (GPSR) is a set of rules that requires consumer products to be safe and our obligations to ensure this.

If you have any concerns about our products, you can contact us on ProductSafety@springernature.com

In case Publisher is established outside the EU, the EU authorized representative is:

Springer Nature Customer Service Center GmbH
Europaplatz 3
69115 Heidelberg, Germany

Batch number: 10732090

Printed by Printforce, the Netherlands